THE
PHARMACIST'S
GUIDE TO THE
MOST MISUSED
AND
ABUSED
DRUGS IN AMERICA

THE PHARMACIST'S GUIDE TO THE **MOST MISUSED** AND **ABUSED** DRUGS IN AMERICA

Ken Liska, Ph.D.

COLLIER BOOKS
MACMILLAN PUBLISHING COMPANY
NEW YORK

COLLIER MACMILLAN PUBLISHERS
LONDON

Collier Books
Macmillan Publishing Company
866 Third Avenue, New York, NY 10022
Collier Macmillan Canada, Inc.

TO THE USER OF THIS BOOK: While every effort has been made to consult recent sources, and while the information herein is believed to be accurate, no warranty is made that each topic is discussed exhaustively, or that product formulas and contents have not changed since publication.

CAUTION: The information contained herein is not to be used for the diagnosis or treatment of any disease or illness, or as a guide for mental or physical health. This book is intended to provide only background information for general health knowledge. Consult your physician if the signs or symptoms of illness appear. Doses given are usually for adults and are for general information only, not as a guide for medication. No claim is made that all trade names for a given substance are included.

Library of Congress Cataloging-in-Publication Data
Liska, Ken, 1929–
The pharmacist's guide to the most misused and abused drugs in
America
Ken Liska.
p. cm.
ISBN 0-02-059340-6
1. Drugs. 2. Drugs, Non-prescription. 3. Designer drugs.
4. Pharmacology—Popular works. I. Title.
RM301.15.L57 1988
615.1—dc19   87-36847
                                                  CIP

Macmillan books are available at special discounts for bulk purchases for sales promotions, premiums, fund-raising, or educational use. For details, contact:

Special Sales Director
Macmillan Publishing Company
866 Third Avenue
New York, NY 10022

10 9 8 7 6 5 4 3 2 1

To Paula Meta

Introduction:
To Dose or Not to Dose

Often one has no choice in deciding whether to take a drug or not. Antibiotics can be crucial in the treatment of infections; dangerously high blood pressure can be controlled with drugs; epilepsy must be controlled, blood clots prevented, and arrhythmias corrected.

But at other times the choice is not so clear. Can conception be controlled by means other than oral drugs? Is a drug always needed for the therapy of depression? Can menopause be managed without exogenous estrogen? Do you need to take a drug to lose weight? Is a muscle relaxant indicated for every sore back? Shall I take a drug to get to sleep tonight? In the areas of OTC drugs, the ads would have us dosing night and day for the rest of our lives. (One ad said, "Take our product and you will be regular the *rest of your life.*")

It is my strongly held belief that Americans are indecently overdosing themselves. I believe that almost all of us could get along with 95% fewer drugs and doses. And this includes prescription as well as OTC (over-the-counter) drugs. A prominent American pediatrician said recently that at least 90% of drugs prescribed by pediatricians are unnecessary and a costly risk to the child who takes them.

There are three reasons we dose too much: (1) Physicians prescribe too often; (2) the ads seduce us with half truths and outright falsehoods; (3) we learned it at home. I have had people come to me with stories of old people in nursing homes receiving 8 to 11 drugs a day, every one prescribed by a physician. One grandmother was so groggy she couldn't walk. Minor tranquilizers are overprescribed; they have become a chemical crutch to many people. Prescription and OTC sleep aids are overrelied on. For the sedentary or for the frail or elderly patient, some type of laxative might be beneficial, but for the healthy person, they are no-win drugs. The more you take, the more reliant on them you become.

Advertising for OTC drugs in some areas is so corrupt that it has become a threat to our nation's health, and this in spite of truth-in-advertising laws recently passed. The worst OTC advertising occurs in the areas of laxatives, cold products, decongestants, shampoos, diet aids, and mouthwash-gargle products. Cases in point: Cold remedies do not cure colds; stomach acid is needed for normal digestion; nasal decongestants act only temporarily; expectorants probably don't work at all; chemical diet aids are poor substitutes for willpower; mouthwashes cannot take the place of tooth brushing and flossing; laxatives, for most of us, disrupt what should be a natural act; colons do not need "cleansing" no matter how vigorously "colon cleansers" are advertised. Half-truths are used, too, as in the ad that tells young women to take a certain antacid because it contains the calcium they need. True, they need calcium, but not at the expense of a serious side effect of alkalinization of the body. Young adults can get all of the calcium they need by eating a variety of foods, including vegetables.

Advertising and formulations for OTC products can be unscrupulous. It is wrong to suggest that acetaminophen can cure fever blisters, help you to sleep, or relieve the inflammation of arthritis. Vinegar does not alter vaginal pH. Alcohol won't neutralize an insect bite. Aloe vera will not help in minor burns or abrasions. Vitamin C will not cure the common cold, grow hair, or remove warts. Aspirin is not a sedative or sleep aid, benzocaine won't cure acne, and boric acid won't cure infections of the eye. Caffeine does not help in rheumatism or fever blisters. Calamine does not neutralize insect bites, nor does camphor act as an effective antifungal or acne treatment. Charcoal will not help control diarrhea, and castor oil is not a skin emollient. Cod liver oil won't heal hemorrhoids. Female sex hormones are not aphrodisiacs, eugenol does not relieve toothache, honey is not an astringent, and kaolin is not an antidiarrheal. Lysine is of no value in weight control. Menthol is not a cough suppressant nor pine tar an expectorant. The ubiquitous peppermint is ineffective in 14 different applications. Shark oil won't cure hemorrhoids. Tannic acid is worthless in 11 different applications. Thiamine will not help you to get to sleep or lose weight. Vitamin E is useless in weight control or acne, and wheat germ oil will not grow your hair. Upon examination, turpentine oil failed in 8 advertised ways, and thymol in 19.

Misconceptions about the use of drugs are unwittingly taught in the home. Is the parent anxious about sleep, bowel movements, acid stomach, indigestion, or state of the sinus? Likely the child will grow to be, too, especially if the medicine cabinet and bedside table are constant reminders.

All drugs have the potential to act as poisons in your body. Some are highly toxic. As you read some of the sections in this book, examine the warnings, cautions, adverse effects, and drug interactions. They show the potential for harm inherent in drugs. And that potential toxicity is predictable when one considers that almost all the prescription and OTC drugs we ingest are foreign to our body. Most are strangers even to this earth, conjured up by a research chemist in a laboratory.

Lest chemists become offended, I hasten to point out that they have given us many valuable agents for waging chemotherapeutic war on disease. But that's not the point. *If* your physician can offer you a drug-free treatment of disease, and respecting the toxicity inherent in chemical agents, you should select the drug-free route.

OTC drugs can contain some potent active ingredients capable of exerting significant side effects. The phenylpropanolamine and pseudoephedrine in OTC products are sold as decongestants and appetite suppressants but in reality are CNS and cardiovascular stimulants. Ephedrine, promoted as an antiasthmatic and antihemorrhoidal, has side effects so serious that authorities now advise against its use. Certain OTC antacids can overalkalinize the system, cause acid rebound, or interfere with the absorption of other drugs. The drowsiness produced by an antihistamine can make the operation of a car or airplane a risky business. Aspirin may be the drug of choice in arthritis, but heavy users know that it has serious side effects. Large doses of caffeine will help one stay awake but may also cause heart arrhythmias or induce psychological dependence. The benzocaine in various local anesthetic products can induce an allergic response.

How can the average person handle the persistent, insidious promotion of drugs in our society, whether it be to the prescribing physician (see the slick ads in the *Journal of the American Medical Association*) or directly to the consumer who is buying over the counter? How can I tell if I really need a drug for my condition? First, examine your mental attitude toward drugs and how you learned it. Do you consider drugs your friends, agents you need to get through the stresses of each day? You may want to reexamine that attitude in light of the fact that a great many happy, healthy people *never take any drugs.* You may find that you take a drug out of habit, not necessity.

Second, discuss with your physician the possibility of a drug-free therapy. If your physician practices holism (an understanding and treatment of the patient's whole life situation), he or she may elect to use nontraditional methods as adjuncts to traditional ones. You may find that your doctor is only too glad to avoid the use of an elective drug.

Third, consider the fact that drugs are typically foreign to your system and that most of them have the potential for significant side effects if not outright toxicity. This is especially true in elderly, debilitated people, or those with preexisting heart, kidney, or liver conditions. It is doubly true in the pregnant woman who should ingest NO drug, drink NO alcohol, absorb NO cosmetic or other external product, and submit to NO X ray unless her physician approves or has so directed.

Last, examine your influence on others. What do members of your family see when they observe your drug-taking behavior or look in your medicine cabinet? What are your examples teaching your children? You may conclude that you do not want to teach them that we need drugs to get to sleep, wake up, digest a meal, defecate, freshen the breath, cleanse the colon, stay young, clear the skin, open the sinuses, relieve gas, or make it through the day!

A

Acapulco Gold. *See* CANNABIS

Accutane. *See* ACNE DRUGS, ISOTRETINOIN

Acetaminophen

Other names: Datril, Tempra, Tylenol, Valadol, Anacin-3, Liquiprin, N-acetyl-p-aminophenol, Panadol

Source: synthesis

Pharmacology: pain reliever, fever reducer

Dose: The usual dose is 325–650 mg (1–2 tablets) every 4 hours for adults and older children, not to exceed 2600 mg (8 tablets) a day. A child of 6 to 9 years is permitted to take no more than 400 mg in 24 hours or to use acetaminophen for more than 5 days unless under the advice and supervision of a physician. Extra-strength acetaminophen tablets contain 500 mg of drug; this higher-strength product makes it easier to overdose.

Acetaminophen is not a salicylate and therefore bears no chemical resemblance to aspirin. But it shares with aspirin the ability to relieve pain (analgesic action) and to reduce fever (antipyretic action). Unlike aspirin, acetaminophen is of no clinical value in the treatment of inflammatory arthritis (though it may be helpful in the pain of osteoarthritis, or degenerative joint disease).

Acetaminophen is derived from aniline, a coal tar chemical. It has gained great popularity since 1949, when it was recognized as the major active metabolite of both acetanilide and phenacetin. An FDA panel has rated it as safe and effective for the relief of pain and the reduction of fever. Acetaminophen lowers fever by a reaction on the brain's heat-regulating center in the hypothalamus. It produces analgesia by elevating the pain threshold. Its advantages over aspirin include the following:

1. It does not cause the GI tract blood loss seen in aspirin use.
2. It does not cause an increased bleeding tendency, so it can be used in tonsillectomy patients and hemophiliacs.
3. As a nonsalicylate, it can be used in the presence of aspirin allergy.
4. It has less potential for causing nausea and vomiting.

Disadvantages to the use of acetaminophen include the following:

1. It is too weak an anti-inflammatory agent to be used in rheumatoid arthritis.
2. It occasionally causes skin rash.
3. In large doses, it is toxic to the liver. Acetaminophen shares this toxicity with all the aniline derivatives. A single dose of 10 g (30 tablets) may result in liver injury. Reversible liver damage has been reported in a 16-year-old after ingestion of a single 5.85 g (18-tablet) dose. A dose of 15–25 g (50–80 tablets) is potentially fatal.
4. Recent reports suggest that even normal doses of acetaminophen may sometimes cause liver damage. For this reason, the maximum adult daily dosage of 4 g should not be exceeded, the duration of use should be limited, and the newer extra-strength formulations should be used with great caution.

Comparative potencies: The ads will tell you "Hospitals prefer Tylenol" and "You can't buy a more potent pain reliever without a prescription." But a recent court decision labeled those claims "false and misleading." Truthfully, there is very little difference in the potencies of aspirin, acetaminophen, and ibuprofen for ordinary aches and pains. But with $1.8 billion at stake in yearly sales, advertisers will stretch the truth as far as possible short of fraud to get you to buy their product. So buyer, beware. Know that ibuprofen can offer some advantages for dysmenorrhea, and acetaminophen is easier on the stomach than aspirin, but overall no one pain reliever offers significant pain relief advantages over the others. Also remember that aspirin, acetaminophen, and ibuprofen can be purchased generically at great savings.

Abuse potential: low

Adverse effects: If you do not exceed the recommended doses for acetaminophen, you probably will not experience any significant adverse effects. However, excessive doses, especially of the extra-strength preparations, can lead to liver damage. The kidney is also sensitive to overdosage. CAUTION: Persons with a known history of liver disease should avoid excessive use of acetaminophen and should restrict its use to brief periods.

Drug interactions: Acetaminophen can increase the effects of concurrently administered oral anticoagulants. Combining alcohol with acetaminophen can increase the poisonous effects of both on the liver. You should either avoid these drug combinations or consult your doctor beforehand.

Acid. *See* LSD

Acne Drugs

Ordinary mild acne is called acne vulgaris. The more severe form, in which inflammation, pustules, and scarring can occur, is termed cystic acne. The incidence of acne is greatest in adolescents, of whom nearly 100% are afflicted. Most acne ends at age 25 or 30. Severe, disfiguring acne afflicts an estimated 500,000 Americans yearly and is the basis for an acne product market that exceeds $130 million a year.

OTC drugs that are used to treat acne include benzoyl peroxide, sulfur, salicylic acid, and resorcinol. These chemicals destroy cells in the top layer of skin, causing the skin to scale, peel, and become somewhat leathery. This relieves pimples and other symptoms.

Isotretinoin (Accutane) is a prescription drug being hailed as the nearest thing to a cure for acne. A chemical cousin of Vitamin A, isotretinoin (13-cis-retinoic acid) has been shown to be highly effective in the treatment of acne. Introduced in 1982, it reduces sebum production up to 90%, producing an almost complete loss of facial oiliness. It does this by shrinking the oil (sebaceous) glands in the skin. Given orally in doses of 1–2 mg/kg daily for 15–20 weeks, isotretinoin is remarkably effective in patients with severe cystic acne that has resisted other treatments. What is more, the drug's helpful effects last for months or even years, whereas the drug itself doesn't accumulate in the body. Of the nation's dermatologists, 90% have prescribed isotretinoin at least once since its release.

Enthusiasm for isotretinoin has been tempered by the discovery that it is a powerful teratogen, probably in the same category with the infamous thalidomide. Nearly 40% of the prescriptions for it are written for young women aged 13 to 19, and FDA records already show that 16 women using Accutane have either miscarried or borne babies with severe birth defects. Fetuses exposed to Accutane develop major malformations at about 25 times the usual rate. It is now clear that isotretinoin must be strictly avoided in pregnancy; before the drug is given to a woman, she should be tested for pregnancy. People taking Accutane should not donate blood. One major adverse reaction to Accutane is cheilitis (drying and inflammation of the lips).

There is a theory that the spurt of male sex hormone at puberty is the cause of acne and that taking female sex hormone (estrogen) should therefore relieve symptoms. This is the reason oral contraceptives (with estrogen content) are used in this dermatological condition. Since estrogen use is statistically implicated in blood clot formation and since pubescent males are not good candidates for estrogen therapy, it would seem wise to examine carefully the risk/benefit ratios in this treatment and to consider alternatives.

Relief of acne symptoms is possible in some cases using ultraviolet (UV) radiation from either sunlight or sunlamps. Here again, the skin toughens and tends to peel, reducing redness and pimple formation. Wise use of UV light is a must! Never allow the high-energy radiation to enter your eyes; wear protective goggles when sitting under a sunlamp. Do not expose your skin for too long. Remember: True UV light is invisible to the human eye; we may not see it, but it certainly is there.

See also ISOTRETINOIN

Actifed. *See* PSEUDOEPHEDRINE

Adam. *See* MDM

Addiction

In the classical medicolegal sense, addiction is a drug-induced change in the physical state of a person such that the continued presence of the drug is now required for normal functioning. Further, upon abrupt termination of the drug, the addict suffers through a physical crisis, of varying degree, known as a withdrawal syndrome (or abstinence syndrome). The withdrawal crisis can be ended at any time by readministering the drug. In this definition of addiction, there is always development of tolerance to the drug, so that ever-increasing doses of it must be taken to get the desired effect. Classical examples of addictive drugs are alcohol, heroin (and all opiates and opioids), barbiturates, and Valium (and other benzodiazepines).

Drug dependence is a modern, more encompassing term that applies to all situations in which users develop a drug reliance, either physical or psychological (psychic), and take their drug on a continuous basis to experience its effects or to avoid the discomfort caused by its absence. Physical withdrawal and tolerance are not necessarily part of drug dependence. Amphetamine-dependent persons can develop a great tolerance to their drug but do not necessarily experience a typical withdrawal syndrome. Their dependence is psychological in nature, but withdrawal can be so serious as to require medical supervision. We can develop a great dependence on and tolerance to caffeine, but we would not classify caffeine as physically addicting, although abstinence can produce some physical symptoms such as headache.

Development of reliance on a drug, whether physical or psychic, depends in large measure on frequency of dose, size of dose, and route of administration. For most drugs, the intravenous route is the most likely to induce reliance. This means that you should try to avoid prolonged use of an elective drug (that is, no longer than a few days or a week at the most). Avoid large doses, especially if taken by intravenous injection. Be all the more careful if you are taking barbiturates or other sedatives, tranquilizers, or narcotic analgesics.

Chemical dependency, yet another term, is synonymous with drug dependence and emphasizes the chemical nature of the ingested substance (as opposed to a prescription drug, plant alkaloid, or OTC preparation). However, everything in our lives is chemical—air, food, drugs—so this term seems a little redundant.

Where to get help: Many communities sponsor agencies that assist the addict or recovering addict. Examples of such agencies are Alcoholics Anonymous, Narcotics Anonymous, Pill Addicts Anonymous, and Cocaine Anonymous. You can call a cocaine hotline (800-262-2463) for help. Therapeutic communities use live-in social dynamics to change social behavior. Synanon, the prototype therapeutic community, was followed by Daytop Village, Phoenix House, Gateway House, Family Awareness House, Marathon House, and the Odyssey houses in Manhattan. Consult your telephone book under Drug Abuse Information, Narcotics Anonymous, or local, state, or federal listings.

Adverse Reactions to Drugs

There is no drug that does not produce some adverse reaction or undesirable side effect, whether it is barely significant or of tragic proportions. And adverse reactions are to be expected, since almost all drugs are chemicals foreign to the body. Relatively few drugs—such as epinephrine, norepi, L-DOPA, dopamine, growth hormone, and insulin—are also found naturally in the body, whereas all of the opiates, major and minor tranquilizers, antihypertensives, anticoagulants, alkaloids, antibiotics, and diuretics either come from plants or microorganisms, or are prepared in the laboratory as novel, synthetic chemicals foreign to our body. Actually, it is surprising when a new, important drug does not have some significant adverse effect. For convenience, adverse reactions can be grouped as follows:

Drug allergy: To be allergic to a drug means that one reacts to a dose of the drug in an abnormal, unexpected, and unpleasant way, typically with skin rashes, fever, painful joints, or difficulty with breathing resembling an asthmatic attack. Moreover, to be allergic means that we have produced antibodies to the drug, either over long exposure or after brief use. The allergy can be mild or serious enough to threaten life. It is difficult to predict who will be allergic to what drug, but there are some clues: Penicillin is notorious for producing allergies; salicylates, including aspirin, are well known to cause adverse reactions ranging from skin rash, kidney damage, and changes in blood cells to severe asthma, shock, and even death. Asthma itself is a predisposing factor in drug allergies, and about 20% of asthmatic children react to aspirin with breathing difficulties that begin about an hour after exposure to the drug. If you have a history of drug allergies, make the fact known to anybody who is treating you for any illness. Drug fever is an increase in body temperature that typically appears a week after the drug is started, continues as long as the drug is taken, and can be low-grade or very high. Drug fever, which may or may not be accompanied by other symptoms, can be caused by many drugs, but a few common offenders are antihistamines, barbiturates, penicillin, and the sulfonamides.

Anaphylaxis (anaphylactic shock): This describes a very serious, acute, and intense allergic reaction to a dose of a drug in which itching, nausea, cramps, diarrhea, and nasal congestion can occur, possibly followed by constriction of the windpipe, shortness of breath, and sudden loss of consciousness. Anaphylaxis is a medical emergency, and help must be sought at once. Call your doctor or get the person to a hospital without delay. Even a small dose of a drug to which we have become sensitized can cause the massive release of histamine that accounts for all these adverse effects. Anaphylactoid reactions have happened in people being treated with small, daily doses of allergens, as in hay fever therapy. It is the same type of serious reaction seen in people allergic to bee or wasp venom. Epinephrine (adrenaline) is an emergency antidote for anaphylaxis, but it must be administered quickly.

Drug hypersensitivity: To be hypersensitive to a drug can

mean one of two things: Either you have developed an allergy to it, or you react as expected but in an exaggerated manner. We know of some women who develop a full facial flush after even one small drink of alcohol. Caffeine can keep some people awake all night but not affect others. Response to street hallucinogens is highly individual and subject to set and setting. Manic-depressives will show different sensitivity to drugs depending on their mood, as can those who are influenced by circadian rhythms. To become tolerant to a drug means that one has *lost* sensitivity to it. A woman may be hypersensitive to one brand of birth control pill but do very well on another. People can be cross-hypersensitive—that is, their hypersensitivity to one drug automatically makes them sensitive to another. This explains the warning on ibuprofen (Advil) labels to avoid use if you are allergic to aspirin. The cross-sensitivity between ibuprofen and aspirin was initially unexpected because the two drugs are not related chemically. However, in the field of allergy, the unexpected can sometimes be expected.

Drug idiosyncrasy: In an idiosyncratic response to a drug, either no effects are produced from large doses of the drug, or the person responds in an altogether unexpected way. For example, some people become belligerent under the effects of the tranquilizer Valium. Given the CNS depressant morphine, some patients become highly agitated. Some hyperactive children calm down when given amphetamines. It is impossible to predict drug idiosyncrasies.

Photosensitization: Some drugs can sensitize the skin so that brief exposure to the ultraviolet rays in sunshine can result in mild or extreme reddening, inflammation of the skin, or even sloughing off of dead skin tissue. Again, no one can predict which drugs will photosensitize, but it is well known that the major tranquilizers such as chlorpromazine and haloperidol are capable of causing this adverse reaction. Some antibiotics are photosensitizers, too, as can be some antihistamines, barbiturates, procaine-type local anesthetics, nonsteroidal anti-inflammatories, salicylates, sex hormones, thiazide diuretics, and sulfonylurea antidiabetics.

Side effects: By the time a new drug has passed through all the tests required before the FDA will approve it, many of its actions beyond those of the major, intended responses are also known.

We call these its side effects. A multitude of side effects are possible with drugs and can be related to the size and frequency of dose, absence or presence of food in the stomach, prior exposure to the drug, tolerance that might have developed, current administration of interacting drugs, set of the mind (placebo effect), and possible drug sensitivity or idiosyncrasy. A few of the common side effects to drugs are: nausea, vomiting, skin rash or flushing, dizziness, and postural hypotension (feeling dizzy upon abrupt standing). Other side effects are much less common. The heart can be affected: tachycardia (too fast a beat); arrhythmia (irregular heartbeat); bradycardia (too slow a beat); hypertension (blood pressure too high); vasoconstriction; or vasodilation. In agranulocytosis, white blood cells are destroyed; in aplastic anemia, red blood cell production is altered. Some drugs can cause cataracts of the eye. Oral contraceptives can alter the pigment in the skin or cause retention of body water.

What you can do to reduce your risk: Usually there is no way to predict the first allergic or hypersensitive reaction to a drug. However, once you know or suspect sensitivity, take every precaution by notifying doctors, nurses, and hospital staff that you have a drug sensitivity. Usually you will be asked about drug allergies before anything is administered to you. Highly allergic persons with known risks can carry with them at all times a hypodermic syringe loaded with epinephrine. Consult your physician about this.

Afrin

Other name of active ingredient: oxymetazoline
Source: synthesis
Pharmacology: nasal decongestant
Dose: For adults and children 6 years and older, spray 2–3 times in each nostril twice daily morning and evening. Do not use this product for more than 3 days.

Advertised as a nasal shrinker, this 12-hour nasal spray contains the sympathomimetic oxymetazoline in 0.05% solution. It is also sold as drops.

Nasal congestion is to be expected with most head colds. It is uncomfortable but temporary, and it will disappear shortly if left alone. The problem with using a nasal shrinker (or decongestant) is that the relief is short-lived, and another dose must be taken. What is worse, in some users a rebound congestive effect occurs in which the congestion is more acute after the drug's effects wear off. This necessitates another dose of shrinker, and another, until one is tempted to sniff all day long, but with no real relief. It is also important to note that the oxymetazoline or other shrinker drug can have adverse effects upon the brain or heart. Sensitive users might find it hard to sleep at night. The conclusion can be reached that since shrinkers work only briefly and can have serious side effects, it is better to avoid them in the first place.

NOTE: An infection can be spread from one person to another if a spray device is shared.

Misuse potential: medium

Adverse effects: When used as directed, oxymetazoline probably will produce no significant adverse effects in most users. Excessive or prolonged use (longer than 3 days) is to be avoided because of the possibility of producing rebound nasal congestion and rhinitis.

Drug interactions: Users of Afrin should avoid concurrent ingestion of epinephrine or other stimulants to avoid overstimulation of the heart and blood pressure. Concurrent use of Afrin and Parnate, Nardil, or other monoamine oxidase inhibitor drugs is to be avoided for the same reason.

AIDS Drugs

The infectious organism in Acquired Immune Deficiency Syndrome (AIDS) is a virus, and that makes a great difference in the way this disease can be treated. Bacterial infections are far easier to treat because bacteria grow and multiply outside body cells, where drugs can act to inhibit or kill them with less chance of damaging the host. A virus is little more than a piece of protein with reproducing capability, and it must remain inside a host cell if it is to multiply.

Inside a host cell a virus like AIDS can take over and damage vital functions. AIDS is the first infectious disease in history to take over the body's immune system, crippling our defenses, permitting a host of other pathogens to take over and run wild. These so-called opportunistic infections are the actual cause of death.

At present, there is no cure for AIDS (despite the paperback with the title *Cure AIDS the Natural Way*). There is as yet no vaccine, nor even a really satisfactory treatment for AIDS. However, a prodigious research program is under way to discover drugs that will inhibit viral replication, and dozens of potential treatments are in clinical and preclinical study.

To date the most successful treatment (not cure) of AIDS and AIDS-related complex (ARC) is the drug AZT, now marketed commercially by Burroughs Wellcome as Retrovir. Retrovir does not kill viruses, but it does mess up their replicating machinery. It is a bogus molecule that is so similar to a critically needed viral substrate that the key viral enzyme mistakes it for the true substrate and as a result is inhibited by it. This confounds the whole replication process, and the virus stops growing. Think of it this way: A car is built with an engine that fits under the hood perfectly but has no cylinders. That car isn't going anywhere. Neither is the virus.

AZT works, and patients get to feel a great deal better—at first. But later, the serious adverse effects of this drug can appear. AZT damages the blood-forming organs of the body, causing anemia and a deficiency of white blood cells. In many cases the anemia is so severe that the drug must be discontinued. AZT treatment can cost as much as $12,000 a year per patient.

Scientists have prepared other "false building blocks," some of them similar to AZT. Dideoxycytidine (DDC) is a very potent inhibitor of viral replication. Ribavirin, a triazole nucleoside, shows promising activity in AIDS patients. It is sold as Virazole in Mexico and 30 other countries but is not licensed in the United States. Many others have been synthesized and are in preclinical trial. Realistically, the "false building block" approach will often suffer from the fact that these drugs are not selective and may damage normal body processes as well as those of the virus.

The AIDS virus hibernates in the body; the vast majority of people infected show no clinical signs of disease. Thus there is a need to develop drugs that will prevent the development of full-blown AIDS or ARC in these people. Such drugs are not now available. We do not know if they would have to be taken for the life of the infected person.

Yet another approach to treatment of AIDS deals with restoring the patient's damaged immune system. Scientists are now investigating immune modulators—drugs that can reinvigorate the weakened immune defenses. Ampligen and interleukin-2 control the body's production of interferons. Isoprinosine and alpha-interferon have been investigated for their immunostimulatory effects.

Since chemotherapy has not solved the problem of AIDS, vaccine development is being given high priority. But here again, there are formidable obstacles. The AIDS virus shows great genetic variability. Many strains are known, each with a different outer protein coat, which is the part usually recognized and attacked by the antibody in the vaccine.

Because we have no cure for AIDS, either with a chemical or a vaccine, prevention is the only effective attack on this disease.

CAUTION: The threat of AIDS and its consequences can motivate the patient to try any drug or substance purported to be a cure. Unscrupulous dealers have treated AIDS victims with snake venom, enemas, umbilical cord extract, thymus extract, acupuncture, garlic, herbs, megadose vitamins, laetrile, amino acids, zinc, selenium, meditation, and colostrum. One AIDS patient is taking 100 pills a day; another spends $600 a month for food supplements, $300 for acupuncture sessions, $250 for colonics, and $500 for sessions with a holistic doctor. Many patients travel to Mexico to purchase investigational drugs not sold in the United States. Although no one can advise a patient whose life is threatened to avoid a purported cure, one can advise that unscrupulous dealers are all too ready to fleece the easily deceived with bogus alternative therapies. Furthermore, we must consider the power of the placebo effect when we take any drug (see the section on placebos).

Alcohol

Other names: ethanol, ethyl alcohol, grain alcohol, C_2H_5OH, distilled spirits

Sources: fermentation, synthesis

Pharmacology: CNS depressant, teratogen, gastric irritant, diuretic, hypoglycemic, peripheral vasodilator

Dose: variable

Ethyl alcohol is the most important drug in the United States on the basis of its use, abuse, and impact on society. It must be carefully distinguished from its poisonous chemical cousin methyl alcohol (wood alcohol).

A common misconception about ethyl alcohol is that it is a stimulant. It isn't. Alcohol depresses the central nervous system (CNS), brain, and spinal cord in all quantities and will induce coma if the blood alcohol concentration (BAC) is high enough. It is the release of inhibitions mediated by alcohol that makes one feel like a better player, lover, or driver of fast automobiles.

Another misconception is that alcohol will keep you warm in cold weather. If you drink in cold weather, alcohol will dilate blood vessels in your skin, causing a feeling of warmth as peripheral circulation increases. However, heat loss from the skin was just what your body reflexes were trying to avoid, and you will ultimately find yourself *colder* than you would have been without alcohol.

A "100 proof" gallon is 1 gallon of 50% alcohol (the proof is always twice the percentage). Hence, 86 proof whiskey is 43% strength. Alcohol is very cheap to make, costing only pennies a pint. We pay so much for alcoholic beverages because of the federal taxes and the cost of advertising. Denatured alcohol is not taxed; neither is it fit to drink, for poisons have been added to make sure it is employed in external-use-only preparations. There is no way the layperson can remove the denaturants.

Pharmacology: Besides being a CNS depressant, alcohol is a teratogen. That means it can cause birth defects. Indeed, the fetal alcohol syndrome (FAS) is now very well known and widely discussed. Women: If you are pregnant, do not drink, for even one drink increases the risk of birth defects. Above all, avoid binge drinking during your pregnancy.

Alcohol irritates the lining of the stomach. The uncomfortable, nauseous, sour feeling we have the morning after a night of drinking probably is due to alcohol's effects on the stomach. As most of us have discovered, we can reduce these effects by eating some oily or fatty foods before we begin to drink. As regards to hangover remedies, there are no certain cures. Perhaps replacement of lost fluids and vitamins B and C would help.

Alcohol is a diuretic. That means it increases the flow of urine. Of course, if we consume a lot of fluid as part of the beer or wine, we are going to experience copious urination anyway. Nonetheless, alcohol can cause some body dehydration.

Alcohol is a hypoglycemic. That means its use causes a fall in blood sugar. This effect can be minimal or so severe that unconsciousness results. Any unconscious person smelling of alcoholic beverage should be checked for hypoglycemia.

There is evidence for a strong link between chronic alcohol use and cancer of the mouth, pharynx, larynx, and esophagus. Although no proof exists that alcohol alone is a carcinogen, combining alcohol with other toxic substances (tobacco, nitrosamines, asbestos, polycyclichydrocarbons) appears to result in increased susceptibility to cancer.

BLOOD ALCOHOL ESTIMATION CHART*

Estimated % of Alcohol in the Blood by Number of Drinks in Relation to Body Weight

Number of Drinks*	Body Weight in Pounds								
	100	120	140	160	180	200	220	240	Not Legally Under The Influence
1	.04	.03	.03	.02	.02	.02	.02	.02	
2	.08	.06	.05	.05	.04	.04	.03	.03	
3	.11	.09	.08	.07	.06	.06	.05	.05	
4	.15	.12	.11	.09	.08	.08	.07	.06	
5	.19	.16	.13	.12	.11	.09	.09	.08	Driving Ability Impaired
6	.23	.19	.16	.14	.13	.11	.10	.09	
7	.26	.22	.19	.16	.15	.13	.12	.11	
8	.30	.25	.21	.19	.17	.15	.14	.13	Definitely** Under The Influence
9	.34	.28	.24	.21	.19	.17	.15	.14	
10	.38	.31	.27	.23	.21	.19	.17	.16	

*One drink is 1 Oz. of 100-proof liquor,
        12 oz. of beer, or
        4 oz. of table wine.
Subtract .015 for each hour of drinking.
**In California, the legal BAC limit is 0.10%

Copyright © Public Safety Department, Automobile Club of Southern California. Used by permission.

The more one drinks, the higher the BAC, as shown in the above table. Of course, food in the stomach delays alcohol absorption, and liver metabolism lowers BAC. The average 150-pound person can metabolize about ⅔ ounce of straight whiskey or 8 ounces of beer per hour. Women generally have more body fat and less body water than men and consequently will show a higher BAC with the same dose of alcohol adjusted for body weight. In most states, a BAC of 0.1% (0.1 g in 100 ml of blood) is legal evidence of intoxication. However, we know that driving skills start becoming impaired at 0.04% and that many people are driving on public roads with BACs of 0.3 and even 0.4%! Laws in most states specify that if you are driving on a public road, it is deemed that you have automatically given your consent to a chemical test for alcohol (implied consent laws). Usually you have a choice of giving a breath, blood, or urine sample. Breath alcohol analysis is most often employed and is quite accurate. Urine testing is least often used and is by far the least accurate.

The role of genetic factors—that is, the heritability of alcoholism—has been studied intensively for 80 years. Researchers are now convinced that heredity plays a role in determining individual differences in susceptibility to alcoholism. They believe that a genetic influence is identifiable in 35–40% of alcoholics and alcohol abusers and that both men and women are affected. If there are alcoholics in your family, you are at greater risk. By the way, the only drug for which an inherited predisposition has substantial scientific support is alcohol.

Alcoholism: If I drink more than a couple of cans of beer a day, or if I get drunk only once a month, or if I drink before noon, am I an alcoholic? Of the many definitions of the complex illness of alcoholism, the following probably would be accepted by most authorities:

> Alcoholism is a complex disease or behavioral disorder characterized by preoccupation with obtaining alcohol and loss of control over its consumption to the extent that use exceeds the ordinary social drinking habits of the community. It is chronic, progressive, and associated with poor health, physical disability, and impaired interpersonal relations or economic functioning.

Note that this definition does not specify the quantity of alcohol consumed as a criterion of alcoholism, for there is too much variation in how much alcoholics drink. The person who drinks only on weekends, or drinks only beer, may fit the definition as well as the person who starts drinking bourbon every day at 7:00 A.M.

Tolerance to alcohol and physical dependence to it develop all too easily. There are about 12 million alcoholics and problem drinkers in the United States. Abrupt withdrawal from alcohol causes a syndrome similar to that for barbiturates: tremors, sweating, nausea, diarrhea, hallucination, disorientation. In severe cases, delirium tremens (DTs, rum fits) may occur, with possible convulsions and cardiovascular collapse. In alcoholic blackouts, the person appears to be behaving normally, but later, when sober, has no memory of what he or she did or where he or she went. Professionals now view alcoholism as a disease and the alcoholic as a physically sick person. To overcome the alcoholic's typical denial of his or her problem, the technique of intervention has been devised. Intervention is a procedure in which close family members, friends, clergy, and employers all together confront the alcoholic with facts about his or her illness in a loving, receivable, undeniable manner.

Alcoholics Anonymous (AA), an organization that has a record of success in changing the long-term behavior of problem drinkers, uses the self-help, semireligious approach, with regular participation in meetings and mutual aid among members.

Alcohol-drug interactions are real and potentially dangerous. The most notorious is the alcohol-barbiturate interaction in which the two drugs act synergistically (2 + 2 = 5) to depress respiration and threaten life. Never combine alcohol with barbiturates. Because alcohol depresses respiration and the CNS generally, its combination with any other CNS depressant (antihistamine, tranquilizer, narcotic analgesic) can result in dangerous additive effects. Here is a summary of alcohol-drug interactions:

- Barbiturates. Synergism with alcohol can be lethal.
- Analgesics. Aspirin, for example, can combine to cause severe stomach irritation.
- Anesthetics. Alcohol can potentiate the effect of an anesthetic.
- Oral anticoagulants. Alcohol enhances their metabolism and so reduces their effectiveness.
- Anti-high blood pressure drugs. When combined with alcohol, they can lower the blood pressure too much.
- Anticonvulsants. Alcohol speeds up the metabolism of dilantin, for example.
- Oral hypoglycemics. This combination can produce dizziness and nausea.

- Antihistamines. Patients can become overly drowsy and have an accident
- Minor tranquilizers. The bad effects on performance, skills, and alertness are increased.
- Major tranquilizers. Phenothiazines can combine to produce possibly fatal respiratory depression.
- Narcotics. Alcohol intensifies the CNS-depressant action.

Alcohol in combination with any drug that has a depressant effect on the CNS represents a special hazard to health and safety and sometimes to life itself. The drug adds to the normal depressant effect of alcohol, further depressing the nervous system, which regulates vital body functions. There is a second type of drug interaction with alcohol. Alcohol can sometimes interfere with the same liver enzymes that metabolize other drugs, and can result in alterations in the rate of metabolism of the other drugs. Depending on the drug and whether the person is an occasional or a chronic drinker, the effects of these other drugs can be either increased or decreased.

Alka-Seltzer

There are three forms of Alka-Seltzer on the market:

1. Alka-Seltzer Effervescent Antacid contains sodium bicarbonate (baking soda), potassium bicarbonate, and citric acid. In the presence of water, these dry chemicals react to release carbon dioxide gas. While sodium bicarbonate is a potent antacid for treating symptoms of occasional indigestion, it is contraindicated for longer than two or three days' use because prolonged use can lead to systemic alkalosis (the body becomes too alkaline). Theoretically, this could result in a rebound effect in which the stomach secretes even *more* acid. Second, daily use of sodium bicarbonate as an antacid may result in sodium overload. For sodium-watchers this could be a serious problem. (Alka-2 Chewable Antacid Tablets contain calcium carbonate instead of sodium carbonate.)
2. Alka-Seltzer Effervescent Pain Reliever and Antacid with Specially Buffered Aspirin contains 324 mg of aspirin per dose, plus sodium bicarbonate and citric acid. The manu-

facturers state that this product when mixed with water produces only a slightly acidic solution (pH between 6 and 7) and therefore will not irritate the lining of the stomach the way unbuffered aspirin notoriously does. CAUTION: Adults to age 60, do not exceed 8 tablets in 24 hours; above age 60, 4 tablets in 24 hours; children 6 to 12 years, do not exceed 4 tablets in 24 hours; children 3 to 5 years, 2 tablets in 24 hours. Do not use if you are allergic to aspirin or are on a sodium-restricted diet. This same product is also sold in an extra-strength form containing 500 mg of aspirin—probably an unwise choice, since aspirin is the potential stomach irritant.

3. Alka-Seltzer Plus Cold Tablets contain phenylpropanolamine (PPA, a nasal decongestant), chlorpheniramine (like all antihistamines, considered to be ineffective in preventing or aborting the common cold), and aspirin. This is another of the many "shotgun" products for colds, and while there are only three ingredients in this product, the criticism is still valid: Most cold sufferers will be overmedicated with this product. It is wiser to treat individual symptoms with individual drugs (or with nondrug approaches as the occasion arises). Persons allergic to aspirin should avoid this product. Note that antihistamines can cause drowsiness, making the operation of a vehicle dangerous.

Adverse effects of antacids: Reliance on an antacid is abnormal, and daily use of them can be dangerous. The acid in your stomach is necessary for proper digestion, and if you have too much stomach acid because of stress or certain foods, it is wiser to correct the cause than to treat with antacids. (Of course, if your doctor has prescribed an antacid for an ulcer or other condition, you will want to follow his or her directions exactly.) Daily or frequent use of an antacid like Alka-Seltzer can possibly cause the body to become too alkaline, a condition in which the stomach tries to produce *more* acid to compensate.

Adverse effects of phenylpropanolamine: Although it is true that this nasal shrinker was designed to have minimal stimulatory effects, it can excite the heart and brain, and some users may discover their heart beating at a faster rate or their mind

stimulated at bedtime after using a preparation containing phenylpropanolamine. You are far better off avoiding Alka-Seltzer
or any antacid or product containing phenylpropanolamine.
See also COLD REMEDIES, ASPIRIN, PHENYLPROPANOLAMINE,
ANTIHISTAMINES

Alka-2. *See* ALKA-SELTZER

Aloe Vera

Aloe vera *(Aloe barbadensis)* is a plant of the lily family that
looks more like a cactus because of its long, spiny leaves. The
juices of many species of aloe have long been used around the
world as cathartics.

For various reasons, including magazine articles and an un-
told number of personal testimonials and anecdotes, aloe vera
has recently become the darling of home remedies, touted for
tooth and gum pain, cuts and abrasions, flash burns, chafing,
sunburn, athlete's foot, fever blisters, poison ivy, poison oak,
joint and muscle pain, arthritis, cobalt radiation damage, and
scar tissue relief.

When leaves of aloe are slit or broken, they yield a gel that
is 99.5% water. This juice, containing carbohydrates and some
20 amino acids, is supposed to have all the healing powers
described in the preceding paragraph. It probably doesn't. In
the case of arthritis, we know it doesn't. One aloe vera ad read:

> Amazing rejuvenation plant melts away painful arthritis at little or
> no cost . . . thousands report spectacular results.

The Arthritis Foundation states that aloe vera is an unproven
remedy and that claims for it as a cure are false and misleading.
The states of California, Florida, and Texas have taken action to
stop misleading ads and improper claims made for aloe vera.

Nonetheless, support for aloe vera continues unabated. One
M.D. wrote the *New England Journal of Medicine* that aloe
helped heal his burns. Research in the Soviet Union and the
United States, it is said, is being conducted on the beneficial
effects of intravenously injected aloe vera juice. Magazine arti-

cles tell us how to grow and cultivate the plant. One article stated, "There's no reason this broad-spectrum natural healer can't become a basic home remedy." Perhaps. But until we have scientific proof from controlled, double-blind studies, we shall retain a healthy skepticism.

Alurate. *See* BARBITURATES

Americaine

This product, sold as a treatment of hemorrhoids, contains the local anesthetic benzocaine and the antiseptic benzethonium (Phemerol). The wisdom of using an antiseptic for simple anorectal discomfort remains to be seen. Some users can develop an allergy to benzocaine. See the section on hemorrhoidal products.

Amphetamines

Other names: Benzedrine, Dexedrine, Desoxyn (methamphetamine), Methedrine, Biphetamine, Paredrine, bennies, dexies, splash, speed, crank, crystal, black beauties

Source: laboratory synthesis (licit and illicit)

Pharmacology: CNS stimulation, bronchodilation, appetite suppression, blood pressure elevation

Dose: 5–10 mg (range: 1–50 mg). Dosage varies greatly with condition and individual patient.

Amphetamines were designed to be similar to adrenaline and to have much the same actions in the body. Indeed, they are sympathomimetic—that is, they mimic the actions that result from stimulation of sympathetic nerves. These actions include:

1. stimulation of the CNS, which leads to elevation of mood and improved concentration, thinking, and coordination
2. delay in the onset of fatigue and the need for sleep
3. increase in blood pressure
4. increase in respiration rate
5. rise in blood sugar levels
6. dilation of bronchi
7. blood flow diverted from internal organs to skeletal muscle

8. constriction of nasal mucous membranes
9. depression of appetite
10. improvement in athletic performance

These ten actions are much like the "fight or flight" response that the body uses naturally to handle stress. Hence we can say that the amphetamines produce an artificial stress in the body.

Amphetamines are prescribed for children with attention-deficit disorders with hyperactivity, and for narcolepsy patients (see section on Ritalin). One of their controversial uses is to control appetite in the treatment of obesity (anoretic action). However, even the manufacturers admit that weight loss of drug-treated patients over placebo-treated patients is only a fraction of a pound per week. The FDA is highly critical of the use of amphetamines in weight control, for it is known that tolerance and a psychological dependence can develop. (One woman built her way up to 30 Desoxyn a day, including a heavy dose on the day she gave birth to a baby.) Also, the benefits usually are short-term and are offset by nervousness, CNS excitation, and other side effects. The Drug Enforcement Administration has criticized the use of amphetamines in "fat clinics." Abrupt withdrawal from amphetamine dependence can result in severe depression, fatigue, increased appetite, and high fluid intake.

People who use amphetamines regularly to get going in the morning, to move ahead in their job, to compete in athletics, or to lose weight may discover that they need drugs like barbiturates to sleep at night. The downers, in turn, enhance the need for more stimulants the next morning; thus a vicious cycle may develop. For a discussion of how long amphetamines can be detected in blood and urine after the last dose, see the section on methamphetamine.

The amphetamines that appear on the street sometimes come from hijacked or otherwise diverted ethical products, but more often from illicit laboratory synthesis. Illicit amphetamines are used as pep pills to delay fatigue for truck drivers or by athletes in highly competitive sports. High doses (100 mg or more) of amphetamines injected intravenously produce a pleasurable euphoric rush or "flash." The most commonly used drug here is methamphetamine ("crystal"). As tolerance develops, the "speed freak" will inject hundreds of milligrams of crystal a day—for days at a time, not wanting to come down off the euphoric high (called crashing). Such an abuser is overactive, irritable, shows defective reasoning and judgment, and may experience irregular heartbeats, liver damage, paranoia, and possible cerebral hemorrhage. There is the possibility of a psychotic breakdown.

Because of their high potential for abuse, all amphetamines are regulated under the 1970 Controlled Substances Act. Severe penalties apply for illegal possession or distribution.

Abuse potential: Amphetamines have a high abuse potential. This is because the user finds the stimulatory effect upon the brain highly pleasureful. Furthermore, when the user discontinues the drug, the resulting depression can be highly stressful. Also, tolerance to the amphetamines readily develops, and the user must take even larger doses to satisfy the craving. The potential for amphetamine abuse is so great that it is wise never to begin their use in the first place. Additional information on use and abuse can be found in individual sections in this book.

Drug interactions: Adrenergic blockers such as Inderal are therapeutically incompatible with amphetamines (that means they work against each other). Concurrent use of antacids such as sodium bicarbonate increases the absorption of amphetamines. The actions of tricyclic antidepressants can be increased by amphetamines. Monoamine oxidase inhibitors and amphetamines are a dangerous combination, for dangerously high blood pressure can occur. Combining lithium carbonate with amphetamines can result in diminished amphetamine stimulatory action. Certain major tranquilizers block the CNS stimulatory effects of amphetamines.

See also DEXEDRINE, METHAMPHETAMINE, RITALIN

Amphojel. *See* ANTACIDS

Amyl Nitrite. *See* NITRITES

Amytal. *See* BARBITURATES

Anabolic Steroids

Other names: Anadrol-50, Clostebol, Deca-Durabolin, Kabolin, methenolone, nandrolone, oxymesterone, stanozolol

Source: synthesis

Pharmacology: Hormones that stimulate the buildup of red blood cells, bones, other body tissues, and appetite. They are related in action to male sex hormones.

Dose: individualized. For aplastic anemia, 1–5 mg/kg of body weight per day, although the usual effective dose is lower.

Anabolism means to build up, and steroids are drugs found in our bodies or made synthetically that have a special kind of polycyclic chemical structure. Hence anabolic steroids are hormonal drugs that induce the buildup of protein tissue and other body tissues associated with nitrogen utilization.

The anabolic steroid Anadrol-50 is prescribed by physicians to treat certain anemias caused by deficient red cell production. Other anabolic steroids are prescribed for postsurgical patients, osteoporetics, or in general for those who need to increase their appetite and body-tissue-building processes. One can easily see, therefore, how weight lifters, football linemen, and others would be motivated to use anabolic steroids to build body mass and gain a competitive edge. Indeed, this practice is now open and widespread.

But do anabolic steroids really work to build bigger and more competitive bodies, or does the accompanying training produce these results? Syntex Company, the makers of Anadrol-50, says their product does not enhance athletic ability; other experts agree. But many athletes and coaches are convinced that anabolic steroids work, and the whole matter remains controversial.

Since the synthetic anabolic steroids are all chemically related to the male sex hormone testosterone, they all have the potential for masculinizing the user. This can manifest itself in males by testicular atrophy (with outside androgen, the testes don't need to produce their own) and in females by deepening of the voice, menstrual irregularities, irreversible male-pattern baldness, enlargement of the clitoris, and loss of body curves. In addition, anabolics are believed to be capable of impairing liver function, causing high blood pressure, dramatically lowering high-density lipoprotein (HDL) levels, and causing prostatic and liver cancer if taken in large doses over a long time.

And athletes do take large doses over lengthy periods. One weight lifter readily admitted to taking 100 mg of oral and injectable anabolics each day while in training (5 to 10 mg a day is the recommended adult dose of Anavar for debilitated patients). Reports from foreign countries suggest heavy anabolic use by athletes, including women.

Hence considerable controversy has arisen over the use of anabolic steroids in sports. Those who favor their use cite the accepted use of birth control pills in female athletes to delay menses until after a meet, and the practice of blood packing, a procedure in which blood is taken from the athlete and then infused back into his or her body just prior to competition. But the International Olympic Committee (IOC) says no to steroids as well as to psychomotor stimulants and narcotic analgesics. The IOC has spent millions of dollars setting up urinalysis procedures designed to detect even traces of 39 stimulants, 12 anabolic steroids, and 20 narcotic analgesics, including codeine. Winners of Olympic events must provide a urine sample within 1 hour of competition. Urinalysis can detect some injectable forms of anabolic steroids months after the last dose. Oral forms have a much shorter half life and disappear from the body more quickly.

Testosterone itself is being used in sports for its anabolic effects, as is human growth hormone. There is no scientific evidence that human growth hormone can improve athletic performance. Drugs such as anabolic steroids are easy to obtain outside the United States. In Mexico they are sold over-the-counter, as much as you want, just like aspirin. Smuggling them into the United States or possessing them without a prescription is a federal offense, however.

The sports-loving public generally agrees that winning a contest with the help of a drug is unfair and that drug use in sports is to be condemned. One opponent of drug use put it this way: The basic nature of a sports contest is to test the natural abilities of athletes against each other. Drugs change that basis. Therefore, drugs have no place in sports. In spite of this belief, drug use continues to be widespread in America and throughout the world.

Abuse potential: There is high potential for abuse of anabolic steroids. Many coaches and individual athletes believe that these drugs will give them a competitive edge, and steroid use is widespread. Some athletes are reported to be taking 30–40 times the recommended dose.

Adverse effects: In women, anabolic steroids can cause a loss of femininity; in men, the testicles can shrink. Anabolic steroids can damage the liver, cause high blood pressure, and induce cancer of the prostate or liver. Winners of athletic contests who are caught with evidence of anabolic steroids in their urine can lose their medals.

See also DRUGS IN SPORTS, STEROIDS

Anacin

Assuring itself a large space on the stores' shelves, Anacin comes in five different variations: regular and maximum-strength aspirin-type, regular and maximum-strength acetaminophen-type, and an acetaminophen children's product.

Regular Anacin is sold as a painkiller, and it makes no sense that it also contains caffeine—a stimulant that can cause sleeplessness, jitteriness, and increased blood pressure. It *does* make sense to reject this type of expensive, heavily advertised product ($4.90 for 100 tabs) for inexpensive generic aspirin or acetaminophen if you want pain relief.

The FDA has ruled that for treating the common cold, caffeine is not safe and effective.

The maximum-strength Anacin products contain 500 mg of either aspirin or acetaminophen. See the sections on aspirin and acetaminophen for the dangers of misusing these types of extra-strength formulations.

Abuse potential: low

Adverse effects: Aspirin can irritate the lining of the stomach, even to the point of causing some blood loss. Peptic ulcer patients should avoid the use of aspirin. Tonsillectomy patients should not take aspirin for pain relief. If you have a history of aspirin allergy or drug allergies in general, consult your doctor before taking aspirin. Acetaminophen is of no clinical value in treating rheumatoid arthritis. Larger doses can damage the liver, so do not exceed the manufacturer's recommended dosage. Read the label.

Drug interactions: See the sections on aspirin and acetaminophen for the drug interactions of these agents.

Anadrol-50. *See* ANABOLIC STEROIDS, STEROIDS

Angel Dust. *See* MARIJUANA, PCP

Anoretics. *See* APPETITE-SUPPRESSANT DRUGS

Anorexics. *See* APPETITE-SUPPRESSANT DRUGS

Antacids

Substances that are capable of neutralizing or destroying acids are given the general name *antacids.*

The public turns to antacids to treat indigestion, acid stomach, or ulcers. A peptic or duodenal ulcer is worsened by the release of hydrochloric acid from the lining of the stomach. However, hydrochloric acid is a physiologically natural and desirable chemical needed in the process of food digestion, and it should not be neutralized unless it is present in abnormally high amounts (hyperacidity).

Indigestion and *sour stomach* are imprecise terms for conditions vaguely described as an uncomfortable feeling in the stomach, a burning pain in the lower chest, gas, belching, or nausea. Although it is most likely that the problem does lie in the stomach (irritated by alcohol, spicy foods, or tension) and that an antacid will help relieve symptoms, it is also possible that a far more serious condition such as heart disease or gallstones is the cause of the symptoms (in which case an antacid is highly unlikely to alleviate the discomfort). This fact makes self-medication with antacids potentially dangerous and has made the FDA critical of the advertising blitz for antacid products. Advertisers would like us to believe that if we feel bloated after a large meal we should take an antacid. But the FDA has found that no product on the market shows evidence of being

safe and effective for this condition. It is inappropriate, therefore, to take an antacid or gas reliever just because you "ate the
whole thing."

A common household antacid is "soda bicarb" (sodium bicarbonate, baking soda, $NaHCO_3$). When mixed with a water solution of an acid (whether it is in the stomach or on a car battery),
sodium bicarbonate quickly neutralizes the acid, releasing bub-
bles of carbon dioxide gas. Occasional use of sodium bicarbonate as a stomach antacid in an otherwise healthy person is safe.
But repeated or continuous use is definitely to be avoided, since
it can result in *acid rebound,* a condition in which the stomach
is stimulated to secrete even greater amounts of hydrochloric
acid in a futile attempt to overcome the alkalizing effects of the
antacid. A vicious cycle can develop with possible habituation
to the bicarbonate. Heart or kidney patients on a low-sodium
diet must avoid the use of sodium bicarbonate.

Acid rebound is also possible after repeated ingestion of the
antacid *calcium carbonate,* found in one of the heavily advertised roll products. Occasional use of calcium carbonate is harmless, but it is a sad comment on the American way of life that
many people are seduced into believing that they need to consume a roll a day of this antacid, week after week. That is
abnormal use and could result in problems such as constipation
and acid rebound. A recent ad for an antacid suggested its use
as a source of calcium for teenagers. Adequate calcium intake
is assured by a proper diet of fruits and vegetables. To depend
regularly on an antacid for one's supply of calcium is wrong
because of the highly abnormal systemic alkalizing effect from
constant use of the antacid.

Antacid products with the word *seltzer* in their name are
highly advertised for relief of indigestion. These products typically contain sodium bicarbonate and an acid such as citric acid,
so that when they are mixed with water they fizz through the
release of carbon dioxide gas. Some also contain aspirin, and this
is what gives the people at the FDA heartburn, for aspirin can
be a stomach irritant, and it makes no sense to include it in a
preparation advertised for *relief* of indigestion.

Aluminum hydroxide, $Al(OH)_3$, is an effective, inexpensive
antacid that does not cause acid rebound and can be used by
low-sodium-diet patients. Unfortunately, it tends to constipate

the user. After this fact was recognized, aluminum hydroxide was combined with magnesium hydroxide (milk of magnesia), a known laxative and itself an antacid. The combination has been very successful, and numerous combination products have been marketed having the approval of medical authorities and consumer groups (see Gelusil, Maalox TC, and Mylanta II in the accompanying table). CAUTION: The aluminum-magnesium hydroxide combination product should not be used by patients with chronic kidney disease because a healthy kidney is needed to handle the challenge to the body's acid-base balance posed by the ingestion of the antacid combination. All things considered, if you can stand the taste of the aluminum-magnesium hydroxide combination product, it is probably your best bet as an antacid.

By the way of summary, the FDA has the following advice on the use of antacids:

1. Unless your doctor approves, don't use any antacid for more than 2 weeks.
2. For occasional use, sodium bicarbonate and calcium bicarbonate antacids are acceptable. For repeated and frequent use, rely on the aluminum and magnesium hydroxide combination type.
3. Low-sodium-diet patients must read the label on the antacid product to determine the sodium ion content.
4. Liquid or suspension dosage forms are more efficacious than tablets, since liquids can more easily coat a larger surface and usually contain more buffering capacity. If you use a tablet, chew it up before swallowing.
5. It is wiser to eliminate the cause of the indigestion than to mask the symptoms with an antacid.
6. If stomach problems persist, give up self-medication and get medical help.

Some antacids are formulated with simethicone, supposedly an antiflatulent (gas reliever). The FDA has concluded that simethicone lacks evidence of effectiveness as an antiflatulent. See the section on simethicone. The following table describes some of the OTC antacids available.

Misuse potential: high. It is all too easy to listen to the misleading advertising and overrely on antacids. Overreliance leads to habituation and compulsive use. This is dangerous be-

Brand Name	Dosage Form	Ingredient or Ingredients	Comments
Alka-mints	Chewable	Calcium carbonate	low sodium
Alka-Seltzer	effervescent tablet	sodium bicarbonate and citric acid	high sodium
Amphojel	liquid	aluminum hydroxide gel	low to medium sodium
Delcid	liquid	aluminum and magnesium hydroxides	medium sodium
Di-Gel	liquid and tablet	aluminum and magnesium hydroxides and simethicone	low to medium sodium
Gelusil	liquid and tablet	aluminum and magnesium hydroxides and simethicone	low sodium
Maalox TC	liquid and tablet	aluminum and magnesium hydroxides	low sodium
Mylanta II	liquid and tablet	aluminum and magnesium hydroxides and simethicone	low sodium
Riopan	liquid and tablet	Magaldrate	low sodium
Rolaids	tablet	dihydroxy aluminum sodium carbonate	high sodium
Tums	tablet	calcium carbonate	low to medium sodium

cause antacids can change the normal acid/base balance of our body, possibly leading to kidney stones in susceptible people. Some antacids are constipating.

Adverse effects: Aluminum hydroxide antacids can cause constipation, while sodium bicarbonate antacids can cause acid rebound. If your doctor tells you to avoid sodium, then you should avoid sodium bicarbonate antacids. The use of antacids for days or weeks can lead to undesirable changes in the acid/base balances in your body.

Drug interactions: There are two ways antacids can interfere with other drugs: by changing gastrointestinal (GI) absorption, or by affecting kidney elimination. Antacids of the aluminum, calcium, and magnesium type can bind to (or absorb) many prescription drugs, thus decreasing their absorption from the GI tract. Examples of drugs that can be bound are: tetracycline antibiotics, digitalis drugs, indomethacin, and chlorpromazine. For other drugs, such as quinidine, the use of antacids can increase blood concentrations or, potentially, their effects. Consult your physician before concurrent use of any prescription drug and an antacid. Proper spacing of doses of antacids and prescription drugs can eliminate possible interactions. Because antacids tend to make the GI tract alkaline, they can cause enteric coated tablets to dissolve faster.

See also MAGALDRATE

Antibiotics

When Alexander Fleming discovered penicillin 60 years ago, he opened the door to a vitally important class of agents we call *antibiotics*—drugs produced by molds or bacteria and capable of inhibiting germ growth (*bacteriostatic* action) or even of killing germs outright (*bacteriocidal* action).

Some widely used antibiotics are the penicillins (such as penicillin G and V, amoxicillin, and ampicillin), tetracycline, erythromycin, streptomycin, bacitracin, neomycin, nystatin, and polymixin B (all generic names).

Antibiotics available to the physician can differ from each other on the basis of the following:

- whether they *inhibit* the growth of bacteria (bacteriostatic effect) or actually kill the bacteria (bactericidal effect)
- effectiveness by the oral route
- the kind of invading germ they will attack (broad-spectrum versus narrow-spectrum action)
- whether or not they are resistant to enzymes causing the destruction of antibiotics

It seems wise to limit the purchase of major antibiotics such as penicillin and tetracycline to prescription only, for indiscriminate and casual use of antibiotics by the laity for every real or imagined illness could well lead to the development of adaptation or resistance in the invading organism. Such resistance develops when insufficient doses of the antibiotic are taken repeatedly or when a sufficient dose is not continued until the conclusion of the infection. These situations can give the germ time to make a supply of enzymes to destroy the antibiotic, or can permit mutant forms of the germ to replace the susceptible strains. Either way, resistance can be a big problem—as seen, for example, in the current difficulty in treating penicillin-resistant strains of the organism that causes gonorrhea. This venereal disease has already reached epidemic proportions, and a crisis could be imminent if resistance continues to develop. Penicillin-resistant gonorrhea first emerged in the Philippines, where even the most potent antibiotics are sold without prescription and where prostitutes regularly take penicillin as a prophylaxis against venereal disease.

Another reason for restricting antibiotics to prescription only is that they can cause serious side effects, and a doctor should be involved if this happens. Some individuals are allergic to penicillin (and to ampicillin, a member of the penicillin group). Life-threatening allergic episodes (called anaphylactic shock) can unexpectedly follow its administration. Then, too, antibiotics can upset the normal balance of microorganisms in the human body, such as occurs in the intestine or vagina, which may lead to serious problems. In women taking broad-spectrum antibiotics, growth of the yeast monilia can result in distressing vaginal itch for which treatment may be difficult. Some of the more mild side effects observed occasionally with penicillin use are skin rashes, upset stomach, irritation of the mouth, and diarrhea.

Viral infections such as the common cold and infectious hepatitis are not curable with antibiotics. It is unwise to try to treat a viral sore throat with an antibiotic. This is the reason your doctor may want to take a culture of your throat before antibiotic therapy is begun. If the culture shows that the infection germ is not susceptible to any antibiotic, he or she will not want to risk drug side effects or the development of resistance. If the culture identifies a susceptible germ, then the doctor can select just the right antibiotic and in the dose and drug regimen that will completely knock out the infection. The patient must remember to take all of the dose prescribed and at the correct time. The aim is not to give the bug a second chance.

It is unwise to self-medicate an infection with leftover supplies of antibiotic because specific illnesses require specific types of antibiotics. Indiscriminate use of a leftover antibiotic may only mask symptoms, thus greatly confusing the situation or even prolonging the morbidity.

The only types of antibiotics the layperson can purchase OTC are the ointment or cream types used to treat infections or external surfaces of the body, plus the nasal spray or lozenge types. It has been questioned whether one can expect any value from topical (surface) use of antibiotics, especially in the nose and throat. Neomycin and bacitracin are the antibiotics most commonly selected for use on the skin.

Drug-drug and drug-food interactions in the antibiotic category are potentially significant. One of the most famous is the negative effect of milk and other high-calcium foods on the antibiotic effect of tetracycline. Calcium ions in the milk or milk product combine chemically with hydroxyl groups in the tetracycline, impairing absorption from the GI tract. Tetracycline is one drug that should not be taken at mealtime.

Besides milk products, antacids such as calcium carbonate, milk of magnesia, and aluminum hydroxide interfere with the absorption of tetracycline. Consequently, such antacids should not be taken to offset possible stomach upset caused by the tetracycline.

Use of tetracycline antibiotics during tooth development may cause permanent discoloration of the teeth. Tetracycline may induce photosensitivity, as indicated by an exaggerated sunburn reaction. Pregnant women should avoid using tetracycline, since damage to the embryo may occur. Tetracycline antibiotics should not be combined with penicillin, since these two types of antibiotics have different mechanisms of action, and combining them reduces their therapeutic effectiveness.

The simultaneous use of an anticoagulant drug with many of the antibiotics may lead to an increased bleeding tendency and even hemorrhage. The reason is that many antibiotics reduce the growth of bacteria occurring normally in the intestine. These bacteria, fortunately, synthesize vitamin K, an important factor in rapid blood coagulation. Their suppression leads to decreased vitamin K synthesis, with consequent increased tendency toward bleeding.

If you discover an old antibiotic prescription in your medicine cabinet and the prescription is in a liquid or suspension form, it's best to throw it out. Many antibiotics, especially in liquid or suspension form, rapidly decompose at room temperature, losing their effectiveness. If you are uncertain, call your pharmacist. He or she is trained to answer questions about the shelf life of drugs.

Misuse potential: medium. The potential for misuse of antibiotics results from attempts to use an antibiotic for a condition other than that for which it was prescribed. If you find an old antibiotic prescription in the medicine chest and take it for a viral head cold, you are not only wasting your time (they don't cure viral infections), you also may be inducing resistance in bacteria that are exposed to sublethal concentrations. Your physician probably will want to culture and identify the invading microorganism before selecting an appropriate antibiotic.

Drug interactions: Some antibiotics, such as tetracycline and erythromycin, do not actually kill bacteria but inhibit their growth so the body's defenses can take over. Other antibiotics, such as Amoxil and Keflex, disrupt bacterial membranes and kill outright. Check with your physician before you combine these two types of drugs, as one may inhibit the activity of the other. Probenecid inhibits the body's excretion of penicillin and cephalosporin antibiotics. For best absorption, penicillins should not be taken with meals; this does not apply to amoxicillin. Some sulfonamides appear to inhibit the absorption of oxacillin from the GI tract.

Antihistamines

Other names: brompheniramine, chlorpheniramine, Chlortrimeton, Dimetane, diphenhydramine, doxylamine, pyrilamine, tripelennamine, Temaril
Source: synthesis

Pharmacology: competitive histamine antagonists

Dose: 2–50 mg depending on the individual product. Use the lowest dose that will give the desired relief.

Histamine is present in all organs and tissues in your body, stored in an inactive form and ready to be released as the result of cell damage or contact with pollen, dust, allergens, or chemicals to which the body has become sensitized. Histamine is a potent and powerful agent; its effects include dilation of capillaries, increased capillary permeability, bronchoconstriction, and increased gastric secretion. Histamine can be the culprit in asthma attacks; ulcers; allergic diseases; sneezing; running of the nose; and itching of the eyes, nose, and throat. There are two types of histamine receptors in the body, designated H_1 and H_2. H_1 receptors are associated with bronchoconstriction and rhinitis, whereas H_2 receptors are associated with gastric secretion.

Antihistamines are synthetic compounds designed to block the action of histamine in body tissues; they do not prevent the release of histamine. They block histamine by preferentially competing for and blocking H_1 or H_2 receptor sites. An FDA panel has found antihistamines to be safe and effective especially in the treatment of allergic rhinitis, but antihistamines were found to have no ability to prevent or abort the common cold. Nonetheless, they are found in almost all OTC cold remedies, where the best they can do is diminish the amount of mucous secretion. If you go to purchase an antihistamine OTC, you will find the generic brands far less expensive than the trade brands, and the corresponding chemicals are the same.

A common side effect of the classical antihistamines is drowsiness—often severe enough to interfere with driving a car or the operation of machinery. (This effect is used deliberately in sleep aids; see that section.) However, the first of a new generation of antihistamines of the nonsedating type is now FDA-approved. Called Seldane, it is an effective antihistamine that is promoted as causing no drowsiness, sedation, or decreased attention time. Seldane (terfenadine) works in the tissues to block histamine, but because it does not readily cross the blood-brain barrier, very little of it can get into the brain and cause sedation. It is available by prescription only.

Misuse potential: high. Because of misleading advertising, many people are led to believe that antihistamines can cure the common cold or hasten recovery. They can do neither, but may provide relief from specific symptoms. If you are uncomfortable, choose a cold remedy that will address your specific discomforts. Avoid the use of colds remedies that contain antihistamines.

Adverse effects: WARNING: Antihistamines must be avoided or used with considerable caution if you are suffering from peptic ulcer, narrow-angle glaucoma, GI obstruction, enlargement of the prostate gland, or bladder neck obstruction. Most of these adverse effects are due to the anticholinergic properties inherent in many antihistamines. The dry mouth, difficulty in urination, and impotence sometimes seen in antihistamine use are also based upon these properties.

Drug interactions: Antihistamine drug interactions are well known. Alcohol combined with antihistamines can cause serious sedation. Barbiturates combined with antihistamines at first cause severe CNS depression; later they nullify each other's actions.

Aphrodisiacs

An aphrodisiac is a sexual stimulant, supposedly capable of exciting one to high sexual desire and performance, hence increasing the pleasure of the sex act.

There probably aren't any true aphrodisiacs, but for hundreds of years many substances have been misrepresented as such. One famous example is "Spanish fly," actually the dried insects of a species of *Cantharis,* from Spain or Russia. Spanish fly is actually a dangerous blistering agent that is an irritant stimulant to the reproductive and urinary organs. A condition of swollen, painful genitals, and ruptured membranes is not sexual stimulation. Spanish fly is not an aphrodisiac.

Alcohol, methaqualone (Quaalude), barbiturates, and other drugs have been touted as aphrodisiacs. Generally, these drugs remove inhibitions and make one *feel* that he or she is a better lover or performer, but this is not true aphrodisia.

There have been reports of a near-aphrodisiac effect produced by L-DOPA, a drug used to treat geriatric male Parkinson patients. Cholestyramine (an anticholesterol drug) has been reported to increase libido. The antidepressant drug trazodone (Desyrel) is known to cause persistent abnormal erection of the penis in a significant number of users; in some, surgery was required to terminate the priapism. Clearly, none of these drugs should ever be taken for their alleged aphrodisiacal effects because of the potential for serious side effects. Yohimbine, a drug from a plant source, has been investigated as an aphrodisiac in males with erectile impotence. See the section on yohimbine.

Appetite-Suppressant Drugs

Our population is overweight by an estimated 1 billion pounds. At the time of our Civil War, the average weight of a 5-foot, 8-inch man between 30 and 34 years was 137 pounds; today he is likely to weigh 170 pounds. To lose weight, many Americans have turned to stimulant drugs. It has been known since the 1930s that amphetamines and other sympathomimetics depress the appetite by stimulating the brain and putting the user into a semiexcited state much like that of a flight-or-fight situation. When we are angry, excited, or fearful, we don't have an appetite, and that is the kind of state these drugs mimic. Hence they are widely used as diet aids, with a yearly U.S. market of over $200 million.

The following table lists 8 over-the-counter diet pills that work by brain stimulation or local anesthesia of the taste buds. PPA stands for phenylpropanolamine.

Most of these diet aids are formulated as timed release and

Appetite-Suppressant Products

Trade Name	Active Ingredient	Cost Comparison per Equivalent Dose
Acutrim	PPA, 75 mg	22¢
Appedrine	PPA, 75 mg (per day)	13¢
Caffedrine	caffeine, 200 mg	16¢
Control	PPA, 75 mg	19¢
Dexatrim	PPA, 75 mg	23¢
Permathene	PPA, 75 mg	18¢
Prolamine	PPA, 75 mg	21¢
Slim Mint Gum	benzocaine (local anesthetic)	11¢

need be taken only once or twice a day. Notice the sameness of these products; nearly all contain phenylpropanolamine in the relatively high dose of 75 mg. A dose of 200 mg of caffeine is also high; sensitive users will experience heart arrhythmias or tremors from that much caffeine.

PPA is a powerful CNS stimulant, and it shouldn't be taken lightly. At higher doses it can cause insomnia, restlessness, nausea, and a rise in blood pressure. One of the public-interest consumer groups states that there is overwhelming evidence that PPA can cause high blood pressure and brain seizures. The PPA manufacturers say there is no reason for concern if the directions are followed. In any event, control of obesity or excess weight by the use of stimulant drugs is not wise, except perhaps in the most intractable cases. It is much better to try to control the reasons for excess food intake, or to encourage exercise. The following table lists antiobesity drugs that are available by prescription only.

Generic Name	Trade Name
benzphetamine	Didrex
diethylpropion	Tenuate, Tepanil
fenfluramine	Pondimin
mazindol	Mazanor, Sanorex
phendimetrazine	Bontril PDM, Dyrexan-OD, Melfiat, Plegine, Trimstat, x-Trozine
phenmetrazine	Preludin
phenteramine	Adipex-P, Fastin, Ionamin

Besides stimulants, there are the following approaches to weight control:

- Bulking agents such as methyl cellulose, psyllium seed, and agar. These drugs supposedly swell up in the water of the GI tract and thus provide satiety; their success has not been established.
- Benzocaine, a local anesthetic that dulls the taste buds.
- Limitation of salt intake and therefore of water retention.
- Psychiatric counseling.
- "Tummy tuck" surgery.

Abuse potential: high. It is easy to get hooked on stimulant drugs used to suppress the appetite. After all, stimulation of the brain and spinal cord is a pleasurable sensation, and when it is ended, our natural desire is to take more drug to reexperience it. What is more, tolerance to these drugs can easily develop, requiring that we take ever larger doses to achieve the same effect. If we suddenly stop taking a stimulant drug, depression can occur. It is very tempting to relieve this depression by taking more of the drug.

Adverse effects: Stimulant drugs, whether over the counter or prescription, can cause restlessness, insomnia, rapid heart rate, and high blood pressure, especially in the elderly or sensitive patient. If you have any kind of cardiovascular disease, see your doctor before taking an appetite suppressant.

Drug interactions: Taken concurrently with other sympathomimetics (such as epinephrine) or with ergot alkaloids, appetite suppressant drugs can cause excessive stimulation of the cardiovascular system. These drugs counteract the actions of antihigh blood pressure drugs. Irregular heartbeat can occur if phenylpropanolamine and digitalis are combined. CAUTION: The use of any monoamine oxidase inhibitor drug simultaneously with phenylpropanolamine or other sympathomimetic is strongly contraindicated.

See also AMPHETAMINES, PHENYLPROPANOLAMINE, SYMPATHOMIMETICS

Aspercreme. *See* COUNTERIRRITANTS

Aspirin

Other names: acetylsalicylic acid, ASA
Source: synthesis
Pharmacology: pain reliever, fever reducer, anti-inflammatory
Dose: 325–650 mg. Each regular tablet contains 325 mg of ASA (the "standard" dose); the recommended dosage for pain is 1–2 tablets every 4 hours, not to exceed 4000 mg (12 to 13 tablets) in 24 hours without a doctor's supervision. Many products on the market now contain the "extra" or "maximum" dose of 500 mg of aspirin.

The fact that we Americans swallow an estimated 19 billion aspirin tablets each year (over 15 tons a day) makes this analgesic (pain-killing), antipyretic (fever-reducing), anti-inflammatory substance one of the most important drugs. Aspirin, methyl salicylate (oil of wintergreen), sodium salicylate, and salicylic acid itself are all chemically classified as "salicylates."

Aspirin is an incontrovertibly effective pain reliever, especially for minor, dull, or low-intensity pain, for headache, or for muscle or joint aches.

Aspirin is the cornerstone in the treatment of rheumatoid arthritis. In fact, most patients' symptoms can be controlled by salicylates alone.

All the salicylates, aspirin included, reduce fever by resetting the brain's "thermostat." Heat production is not reduced, but heat loss is increased by increased blood flow to the skin and by sweating.

Whether you buy the most expensive aspirin or the cheapest generic, it is the same drug, acetylsalicylic acid, and all products must conform to the same standards of purity and effectiveness established by the *United States Pharmacopoeia (USP)*. The unwary purchaser can get royally ripped off in purchasing aspirin. For example, Maximum Strength Ecotrin for Arthritis costs $4.29 (!) for 60 tablets of 500 mg each. You can buy 100 generic aspirin tablets (325 mg aspirin each) for 99 cents and take 1½ tablets for approximately the same dose. You are receiving exactly the same drug.

When you buy aspirin you have the choice of selecting a buffered product—that is, one containing an alkaline chemical that will neutralize (buffer) the acidity of the aspirin when it contacts the stomach lining. Strong buffering reduces the gastric irritant effects of aspirin but does not eliminate them completely. The Food and Drug Administration says there is no evidence that buffered aspirin relieves pain faster than non-buffered aspirin.

Although aspirin is considered a generally safe drug, some things *can* go wrong with aspirin therapy. Because aspirin is an acid, it can irritate the lining of the stomach, even to the extent of causing blood loss. A peptic ulcer patient who takes a lot of aspirin is risking a massive hemorrhage. Tied in with this is the fact that even small doses of aspirin prolong bleeding time in normal people. A single 650 mg dose of aspirin approximately doubles the mean bleeding time for 4–7 days. For the average person this is probably not important, but for the tonsillectomy patient or the hemophiliac, there is good reason to consider aspirin a dangerous drug that must be avoided. (Acetaminophen, a nonsalicylate, does not prolong bleeding time.) Quite remarkably, aspirin and the salicylates have a built-in early-warning system that can tell us when we are overdosing. A ringing in the ears (called tinnitus) signals impending salicylate toxicity. At that point, usage must be stopped immediately.

CAUTION: No painkiller should be taken for longer than 10 days by adults or 5 days by children because persistent pain is a symptom that should not be masked by a drug. Rather, its cause should be found and corrected. Aspirin overdosage can be fatal; death results from respiratory failure after a period of unconsciousness. Before death there is restlessness, incoherent speech, hallucinations, tremors, and convulsions.

Aspergum is an aspirin chewing gum sold for relief of sore throat. However, the application of aspirin (acetylsalicylic acid, remember) to an inflamed throat (assuming significant amounts can even get there) is irrational, for the acidic aspirin can further irritate an already inflamed area. Aspirin chewing gums have no advantage over aspirin tablets for the treatment of sore throats, and they are expensive. I don't recommend the use of Aspergum or any aspirin chewing gum.

Evidence continues to accumulate that aspirin helps to reduce the risk of stroke and heart attack in persons who have had transient ischemic attacks (TIAs, sometimes called small strokes). TIAs, which can indicate an impending stroke, produce the same symptoms as a true stroke but are brief. Studies in both the United States and Canada indicate that 4 aspirin tablets a day will reduce the risk of stroke in men (but not in women). Presumably this effect is related to aspirin's anticoagulant action—its tendency to "thin the blood." The FDA has recommended that aspirin be approved as therapy for TIAs. Another study showed that taking aspirin each day could reduce by 20% your chances of having a second heart attack if you have already had one, and by 50 percent if you are a patient with unstable angina. In a related area, aspirin has been found to reduce significantly the risk of heart attack in men with coronary artery disease.

Some children's aspirin products on the market come in pretty colors and with candylike flavors. Such products are to be deplored because children can perceive them as candy and try to eat large quantities of them.

Abuse potential: low

Adverse effects: Both aspirin and alcohol irritate the stomach lining, and it makes little sense to take ASA to relieve the inflamed stomach associated with a hangover. Aspirin interferes with blood clotting; it can cause bleeding problems in pregnancy or after surgery, whereas acetaminophen does not.

Additional adverse reactions to aspirin occur infrequently but nonetheless are potentially serious. A very small percentage of the population may be highly sensitive (or allergic) to aspirin, suffering rhinitis, hives, shock, or even death from one dose. There is no way to predict who will experience such a reaction to aspirin, although asthmatics are far more susceptible to an attack than are nonasthmatics, especially those with nasal polyps. Salicylates can cause skin rashes, kidney damage, changes in blood cells, and upset stomach. See the section on Reye syndrome for more on aspirin's adverse effects.

Drug interactions: Aspirin interactions are common. Because of its very extensive use, aspirin has an increased chance of interacting with other drugs concurrently being taken. Aspirin combined with alcohol or with an anticoagulant can significantly increase bleeding tendency. Aspirin taken concurrently with oral antidiabetic drugs (such as Orinase or Diabinese) can result in too great a lowering of blood sugar. Aspirin may decrease the antihypertensive effect of Captopril. Aspirin will antagonize the systemic actions of the antiarthritic drugs Anturane and Benemid. If you are taking *any* prescription medication, consult your physician before dosing yourself heavily with aspirin.

See also REYE SYNDROME

AsthmaHaler. *See* ASTHMA PRODUCTS

Asthma Products

In bronchial asthma the air passageways (bronchi and trachea) are hypersensitized and consequently become constricted to the extent that breathing is impaired and wheezing is heard. About 3% of Americans suffer from asthma, most before age 30, and more males than females. Most children with asthma grow out of it by adulthood.

In some families there is a history of asthma; children and parents react to pollen, dust, and other environmental allergens. In others there is no family history, but one sees nasal polyps and often aspirin sensitivity. Up to 10% of asthma patients get a severe attack after taking as little as 300 mg of aspirin. Exercising in cold air can precipitate an attack.

The asthma patient will typically attempt treatment with an OTC drug (discussed below). However, the physician may wish to prescribe a more potent bronchodilator or a greater dose. Prescription bronchodilators include Accurbron, Aerobid, Alupent, Brethine, Bronkephrine, Decadron, Isuprel, Metaprel, Proventil, and Ventolin. Because most of these prescription-only products are sympathomimetics, typically acting as adrenergic agonists, they can produce side effects such as nervousness, a fast heart rate, nausea, sweating, cramps, and central nervous system stimulation. Aerobid and Decadron are anti-inflammatory steroids, not sympathomimetics; they can show adverse reactions, too. Aerobid can cause diarrhea, upset stomach, headache, palpitation of the heart, and upper respiratory symptoms. Decadron's adverse effects include fluid and electrolyte disturbances, muscle weakness, peptic ulcer, increased sweating, and irregular menstruation.

Most OTC bronchodilators contain ephedrine, epinephrine, methoxyphenamine, theophylline, an antihistamine, or a combination of these. The following table lists some OTC asthma products.

Almost all of the sprays or mists on the market contain epinephrine. Although it is true that the FDA has found epinephrine nasal sprays safe and effective for treating acute asthma attacks, it must be noted that epinephrine's effects are brief and its possibility for adverse effects real (see the section on epinephrine). What is more, tolerance to epi's effects can develop quickly and the user may feel compelled to use this potent medication in larger and larger doses. All of this suggests that the use of epinephrine nasal sprays be strictly limited to serious asthma attacks or to occasional use.

Tablets and elixirs constitute the other types of OTC prod-

Trade Name	Dosage Form	Active Ingredient or Ingredients	Rated Safe and Effective by FDA?
AsthmaHaler	mist (inhaler)	epinephrine	yes
Bronkaid	mist	epinephrine	yes
Bronkaid	tablet	ephedrine, guaifenesin, theophylline	no
Medihaler	mist	epinephrine	yes
Primatene	mist	epinephrine	yes
Primatene	tablet	ephedrine, theophylline, phenobarbital, or pyrilamine	no

ucts. The FDA has a lot to say about tablets and elixirs, and it is all negative. These products contain minimal amounts of ephedrine and theophylline, sometimes with an antihistamine or a barbiturate thrown in. The FDA states that while theophylline is often the drug of choice for asthma, the amounts of it found in OTC products are too little to do any good, and larger doses cause serious adverse reactions. Ephedrine, too, can alleviate an asthma attack but can also raise heart rates and blood pressure. In fact, ephedrine has so many serious potential adverse effects compared to the other available bronchodilators that it should no longer be prescribed for asthma.

There is no good medical reason for including antihistamines in an asthma preparation. There is a good reason for excluding them: Antihistamines can dry up respiratory tract secretions, making the asthma attack worse. (Actually, drinking lots of fluids can often help prevent air passageway obstructions.) Similarly, there is no evidence that barbiturates are safe and effective ingredients in asthma products (such as Primatene-P tablets). Barbiturates combined with alcohol can dangerously depress respiration.

In view of the limitations of OTC asthma products, it would appear wise to treat asthma under the guidance of a physician, especially if you are a heart patient, have high blood pressure, or are at risk from other conditions.

See also EPINEPHRINE

B

Bantron Smoking Deterrent

Other name: lobeline
Source: sold over-the-counter
Pharmacology: similar to that of nicotine but less potent
Dose: variable
An FDA panel has found that this product lacks evidence of safety and effectiveness as a smoking deterrent. The supposed active ingredient, lobeline, is obtained from Indian tobacco, which is not the same as *Nicotiana tabacum*. Lobeline bears a chemical resemblance to nicotine and has long been promoted as a substitute for nicotine dependency, but the scientific proof still is lacking.
Abuse potential: low
Adverse effects: Since lobeline's actions resemble those of nicotine, one could expect similar adverse effects (but of less intensity). See the section on nicotine. CAUTION: Do not use this product during pregnancy.
Drug interactions: These are of little significance with minor use of lobeline. Heavy use could result in reduced action of painkillers and tranquilizers.
See also NICORETTE

Barbiturates

Other names: Amytal ("Blue Birds"), Alurate, Nembutal, Pentothal, Seconal ("Reds"), phenobarbital, Tuinal ("Blues and Reds") sleeping pills
Source: synthesis
Pharmacology: central nervous system depressants used as

sedatives and sleep inducers (hypnotics), and anticonvulsants.
Dose: individualized. Depends on patient's age, weight, and
condition, and on the sedative or hypnotic response desired.

Barbiturates are downers. They depress all excitable nerve
tissue, but especially that of the brain and spinal cord. Thus they
can be used in small doses to sedate the excited person or in
larger doses to induce sleep in the insomniac.

Barbiturates can be classified on the basis of how quickly and
how long they act in the body. In most people, short-acting
barbiturates such as Nembutal and Seconal take effect in 15
minutes but act less than 3–4 hours. Phenobarbital, a long-acting barbiturate, takes effect in about 60 minutes but lasts 10–12
hours or more. Pentothal sodium is a widely used intravenous
barbiturate-anesthetic, often employed in dental surgery; its
onset is rapid (30 seconds) and its duration is very brief (10–30
minutes). Elderly or debilitated patients are more susceptible to
barbiturates, and their dose must be reduced accordingly.

Barbiturates are controlled substances legally available by
prescription only. The fast-acting barbiturates are listed in
Schedule II of the 1970 Controlled Substances Act as medically
useful but having a high potential for abuse. The law specifies
stiff penalties for unauthorized possession or distribution. See
the section on controlled substances for a discussion of drug
schedules.

Before the introduction of the minor tranquilizers, barbiturates were the mainstay in the treatment of insomnia. They
work very well but have the disadvantage of reducing time
spent in REM sleep (i.e., they depress dreaming) and of inducing the liver to increase its supply of enzymes that metabolize
barbiturates. Hence tolerance can develop in the long-term
user, and worse, a physical dependency that includes a dangerous withdrawal syndrome. Also, the barbiturates depress respiration. With high doses one can fall asleep and then stop breathing. To make matters worse, the combination of barbiturates
with alcohol is synergistic (that is, they potentiate each other's
actions) in depressing respiration, and more than a few people
have died because they took barbiturates to get to sleep after
a night of drinking. This is one combination you must avoid!
Barbiturates are strong enough to cause death.

Barbiturates are used to control convulsions produced by

brain damage, poisons, tetanus, epilepsy, or toxemia of pregnancy. Phenobarbital is the most useful barbiturate anticonvulsant, being inexpensive, relatively nontoxic, and effective. (Of course, many other nonbarbiturate drugs, including Dilantin, are used to control epilepsy.)

Abuse potential: high. Street use of barbiturates is extensive. They are taken orally or by injection to get "high" (even though they are downers). The user becomes sedated, sluggish in thought and action, but possibly giddy and free from worries. Barbiturates and alcohol produce very similar effects, including loss of inhibitions. Barbiturates are frequently used by thrill-seekers in combination with opiates (a dangerous mixture, since both depress respiration) or as a substitute for heroin when the supply of the latter is cut off. Extended use of barbiturates can easily lead to tolerance, increased dosage, and ultimately physical dependence. To avoid this risk, never use barbiturates for insomnia for longer than a few days. Doctors should not prescribe large quantities of barbiturates. Never keep large numbers of doses around the house.

Adverse effects: Barbiturates inhibit dreaming (dreaming is considered to be a desirable outlet for repressed feelings). They induce the liver to make more enzymes, which in turn hastens the body's destruction of other drugs and chemicals. Tolerance to barbiturates with subsequent dependence can develop. Barbiturates depress the brain and spinal cord; operating a vehicle or machinery while under their influence can be hazardous (in this regard they act much like alcohol).

Drug interactions: Concurrent use of barbiturates and digitoxin can defeat the action of the digitoxin. Short-term barbiturate use combined with alcohol, tranquilizers, or antihistamines may result in oversedation. Isoniazid and monoamine oxidase inhibitors increase the rate of central nervous system depression. Chronic use of barbiturates can stimulate the liver to synthesize enzymes that speed up the body's breakdown not only of the ingested barbiturate but of many other substances as well (tranquilizers, antidepressants, anticoagulants, heart drugs, alcohol, aspirin, and oral contraceptives). In a patient taking a heart drug such as Inderal (a beta-adrenergic blocker), the addition or termination of phenobarbital may necessitate changing the dose of the heart drug.

See also PHENOBARBITAL, SECONAL

Ben Gay. *See* COUNTERIRRITANTS

Benzedrex

Other name: propylhexedrine USP
Source: synthesis
Pharmacology: nasal decongestant
Dose: Two inhalations through each nostril provide about 0.5 mg of drug per nostril. Avoid excessive use.

Benzedrex is sold OTC in the form of a nasal inhaler for the treatment of nasal congestion caused by head colds, sinusitis, and allergies. The active ingredient, propylhexedrine, is not an amphetamine but is chemically similar. It can be considered a sympathomimetic—that is, a stimulant to the heart and brain. It has only about half the pressor (blood-pressure-raising) effect of amphetamine and causes decidedly fewer effects upon the central nervous system.

Each Benzedrex inhaler contains 250 mg of propylhexedrine, theoretically enough for 500 2-snort inhalations. It also contains 12.5 mg of menthol and aromatics.

NOTE: This inhaler loses its potency after 2–3 months' use. Keeping it closed prolongs life.

Abuse potential: medium. One of the side effects common to nasal decongestants is stimulation of the brain. Some people regard such stimulation as pleasureful and continue to use the inhaler for weeks or months. Others can develop a reliance on decongestant inhalers—that is, they find they must use it repeatedly to keep the air passages open. They simply cannot function (breathe) without it. They would have been far better off if they had never used the inhaler in the first place.

Adverse effects: Although it is true that Benzedrex has been designed to have minimal effects on the brain and heart, some sensitive users may discover their heart beating faster or their mind stimulated after using this inhaler. Elderly persons or those with known heart conditions would want to avoid this product.

Drug interactions: With occasional or limited use of this product, little propylhexedrine will enter the general circulation and there will be minimal possibility for drug interactions. Heavy use is another matter. Monoamine oxidase inhibitors potentiate the effects of propylhexedrine. Concurrent use of other stimulants such as epinephrine or appetite suppressants could lead to overstimulation of the heart and brain. If you are using insulin, consult your doctor before extensive use of this product.

See also COLD REMEDIES, SYMPATHOMIMETICS

Benzedrine

Other name: amphetamine
Source: synthesis
Pharmacology: central nervous system stimulant
Dose: 1–10 mg; tablets typically contain 2.5–5 mg each

The effects of Benzedrine, the first amphetamine, were first described in 1930. It is a powerful stimulant to the brain and spinal cord, causing wakefulness, attentiveness, lowered fatigue, mood elevation, increased physical ability, talkativeness, and possible euphoria. Extended use of large doses usually are followed by a serious mental depression when the drug is withdrawn. Overdosage with Benzedrine can cause headache, irregular heartbeat, sweating, dry mouth, vomiting, and intestinal cramps.

Benzedrine is what chemists call a racemic mixture. This means it consists of equal amounts of two mirror-image forms. One of these, the "right-handed" form, is known as Dexedrine (dextroamphetamine) and is 3–4 times more powerful a stimulant than the "left-handed" form. See the section on Dexedrine.

Abuse potential: high. Amphetamine is a powerful stimulant of the brain and spinal cord. Many people find it exciting and pleasurable to use, and they are reluctant to stop its use because of the depression they feel without it. Because of this abuse potential, the use of Benzedrine per se has greatly diminished. However, it is marketed as Obetrol, in combination with dextroamphetamine, for weight control.

Adverse effects: The poisonous effects of amphetamine are usually nothing more than an extension of its usual stimulatory effects on the brain and spinal cord. With doses greater than 10 mg, the user can experience insomnia, restlessness, irritability, headache, palpitation, irregular heartbeat, high blood pressure, dry mouth, vomiting, and abdominal cramps. (Some people will experience these symptoms at lower dosages.) Very high doses can cause convulsions, brain hemorrhage, and death.

Drug interactions: Combining monoamine oxidase inhibitors with amphetamine is risky because dangerously high blood pressure can occur. Amphetamines counteract the effects of heart drugs such as Inderal. Concurrent use of antacids such as sodium bicarbonate increases the absorption and actions of amphetamines. The actions of tricyclic depressants such as Elavil and Tofranil can be increased by amphetamine. Lithium carbonate tends to block the effects of amphetamine, as do certain major tranquilizers. See your doctor before combining these drugs.

See also AMPHETAMINES, SYMPATHOMIMETICS

Benzene. *See* SOLVENTS AND INHALANTS

Benzodiazepines

The word defines a chemical category of minor tranquilizers, the most important examples of which are Valium (diazepam), Librium (chlordiazepoxide), Dalmane (flurazepam), Halcion (triazolam), and Serax (oxazepam). These benzodiazepines are prescribed for the control of neuroses, tension, muscle spasm, alcohol withdrawal, agitation, hallucinations, convulsions, skin rash, and often for insomnia. They have half-lives of up to 72 hours in the body. (The half-life is the time it takes for half a dose to be eliminated from the body.) Benzodiazepines act on specific receptors in the brain but do not depress dream sleep (also called REM sleep) when taken in usual doses. Serax has had extensive use in the treatment of recovering alcoholics, but great care must be taken to avoid a substitution dependency on Serax.

Cross-tolerance can develop among benzodiazepines, meprobamates, barbiturates, and alcohol. (This means that tolerance to any one of these drugs automatically means tolerance to any or all of the others.)

Benzodiazepines have been used to treat PCP intoxication, as anticonvulsants in *petit mal* epilepsy or during a *grand mal* seizure, and as calming agents before surgical anesthesia.

Abuse potential: high. It is too easy to become dependent on benzodiazepines to get to sleep, to calm down, or to handle a stressful situation. Fortunately, they are not acutely toxic. Unfortunately, their safety disarms one into believing that they are harmless drugs that can be taken with impunity.

Adverse effects: Tolerance to benzodiazepines can occur, as can physical dependence if large doses are taken over a long period. Withdrawal from benzodiazepine dependency can be characterized by anxiety, restlessness, tremors, nausea, cramps, diarrhea, muscle spasms, tics, moodiness, confusion, disorganized thinking, racing thoughts, bizarre dreams, hallucinations, paranoia, violence, depression, and possibly *grand mal* seizures. The period of acute withdrawal from benzodiazepines can be as long as 21–28 days (unlike the 72-hour period of withdrawal from alcohol). Some people have died in sedation drug abstinence; it can be a life-threatening situation (see the section on withdrawal). Secondary withdrawal from benzodiazepines commonly lasts for 1.5–2 years. If you have been taking Valium or some other benzodiazepine regularly for months or years, and you wish to stop, consult a physician. You may have become physically dependent on them and you may have to slowly decrease the dose to avoid a significant withdrawal syndrome.

Although benzodiazepines show a lack of effect on heart, skeletal muscle, and other tissues outside the CNS, they have the potentially serious adverse effect of impairing driving ability. Simulation studies show that one 5-mg Valium tablet causes driving impairment equivalent to a blood-alcohol concentration of 0.07% (close to the 0.1% legal definition of intoxication). NOTE: Patients with pulmonary disease should consult their physicians before taking benzodiazepines, as respiratory depression may occur.

Drug interactions: Benzodiazepines, taken together with alcohol, can result in overdepression of the CNS, making driving hazardous (this does not apply to occasional use of small quantities of alcohol). Some Parkinsonism patients receiving levodopa may develop worsening of their Parkinsonism when taking benzodiazepines. Concurrent use of phenytoin and benzodiazepines can result in elevated or depressed phenytoin blood levels. Tagamet may increase the intensity and duration of action of some benzodiazepines. Patients taking digoxin may have an increase in digoxin level when taking benzodiazepines.

See also DALMANE; VALIUM; TRANQUILIZERS, MINOR

Beta Carotene. *See* TANNING PILLS

Birth Defects. *See* ALCOHOL, TERATOGENS

Black Beauties

Other name: Biphetamine
Source: synthesis
Pharmacology: central nervous system stimulants
Dose: 12½-mg capsule (half black, half white), 20-mg capsule (all black). Recommended dose is 1 capsule daily.

Black beauties is the street name for the prescription-only product Biphetamine, which appears as an all-black or half-black, half-white capsule.

The product consists of a 50-50 mixture of amphetamine and dextroamphetamine, both strong stimulants to the brain. See the section on amphetamines for a discussion of the pharmacology.

Abuse potential: high. Prized for its pleasureful stimulatory effects, Biphetamine is an abused street drug. As tolerance to it develops, the user takes ever larger doses and can easily become psychologically dependent on it. When use of the drug is stopped, the resulting depression is very difficult to handle.

Adverse effects: Abusers of amphetamines typically are irritable, hyperactive, show defective reasoning and judgment, and may experience irregular heartbeat, paranoia, and possibly cerebral hemorrhage (owing to very high blood pressure).

Drug interactions: Antacids combined with amphetamines can increase the absorption of the amphetamine into the bloodstream. The action of a tricyclic antidepressant such as Elavil is increased by amphetamines. Never combine an amphetamine with a monoamine oxidase inhibitor, as dangerously high blood pressure may result.

See also AMPHETAMINES

Butyl Nitrite. *See* NITRITES

C

Cafergot. *See* ERGOT

Caffeine

Other names: guaranine, methyltheobromine, trimethylxanthine

Sources: coffee, tea, cola drinks, guarana, kola nuts, chocolate, synthesis

Pharmacology: brain and spinal cord stimulant, heart muscle stimulant, cerebral vasoconstrictor, diuretic, treatment for migraine

Dose: in medicine, 15–150 mg

Americans consume over 100 billion doses of caffeine yearly, or about 5000 tons every 12 months. We get it in coffee (100–150 mg per cup), tea (40–75 mg per cup), cola drinks (40–60 mg per 12 fl oz), No-Doz tablets (100 mg each), Excedrin (65 mg per tablet), and chocolate (20 mg per ounce). It also is found in Anacin, Darvon Compound, Empirin Compound, and Vanquish. You can see that caffeine is a very important tool for manipulating sales of many products in our society. The caffeine obtained by decaffeinating coffee (some 200 tons a year) is used to fortify the caffeine content of some cola drinks.

Caffeine is a significant stimulant of the central nervous system. In 50–200 mg doses it improves alertness, combats fatigue, stimulates the flow of ideas, promotes better physical coordination, and prevents "highway hypnosis." In higher doses it excites the brain and spinal cord, possibly producing tremors, rapid breathing, insomnia, restlessness, irritability, nervousness, and headache. At very high doses (several grams), caffeine causes convulsions. Caffeine is not an effective antidote to alcohol intoxication or hangover because it cannot reverse the depression of the brain produced by alcohol.

Caffeine and the other xanthines (theophylline, theobromine) stimulate the muscles of the heart so that it functions more effectively as a pump. However, in some people this increased myocardial sensitivity shows up as an irregular heartbeat (arrhythmia). Abnormal heart rhythms are likely to be encountered by persons who use caffeine to excess. Caffeine causes constriction of blood vessels in the brain, mild dilation of the coronary arteries, and increased peripheral circulation. Usually a small rise in overall blood pressure is seen.

Caffeine and the xanthines are diuretics. The increase in urine output caused by caffeine, however, is not striking and must be accounted for in part by the increased beverage fluid intake.

Other actions of caffeine include dilation of the bronchi (40% as effective as theophylline), irritation of the stomach, and increased secretion of gastric juices. Peptic ulcer patients should avoid coffee and caffeine.

You may be one of the 1 in 3 coffee or cola drinkers who prefers a decaffeinated brand. A total of 97% of the caffeine in coffee can be removed by treating the green coffee beans with a solvent such as methylene chloride; the beans are then washed, roasted, and ground. However, a tiny amount of the solvent remains, a fact noted by critics of methylene chloride who cite a 1981 study that indicated that methylene chloride is a carcinogen in rodents. Not to worry, says the FDA; the chemical residue is too small to have any effect on humans. Why not switch to the solvent ethyl acetate? says the Center for Science in the Public Interest, for ethyl acetate is just as effective and completely safe. At least two brands of coffee now advertise that they have switched to ethyl acetate in their decaffeination process.

If you prefer coffee with the caffeine left in but want to cut back on caffeine intake, note that automatic drip coffee makers extract more caffeine than do percolators or instant formulas and that brewing coffee twice as long doubles the quantity of caffeine released.

Regarding medical uses, caffeine is prescribed in combination with ergot to treat migraine headaches (Cafergot). Marketed by Sandoz, Cafergot contains ergotamine tartrate and caffeine and is available as suppositories for the patient whose migraine is accompanied by nausea and vomiting. CAUTION: Ergotamine tartrate is a potent vasoconstrictor, to be used only under the continuing strict supervision of a physician.

Abuse potential: low

Adverse effects: Persons who drink 10 or more cups of coffee a day (approximately 1 g total of caffeine) may develop caffeinism, a syndrome in which anxiety, irritability, headache, muscle twitching, and insomnia occur. In one recorded case, a 39-year-old housewife drank 15–18 cups of coffee a day. She had developed a considerable tolerance. Withdrawal from caffeine dependence resulted in restlessness, irritability, headache, shakiness, inability to work effectively, and lethargy. A college woman was ingesting 4 No-Doz tablets and a 6-pack of Cola beverage each day; she had lost 15 pounds on this regimen. Each time she tried to stop the caffeine cold turkey, she developed severe headache, shakiness, irritability, and nausea. A single 12-fl-oz can of diet cola would relieve her withdrawal symptoms.

There are 2 million to 6 million Americans who are afflicted with panic attacks: heart palpitations, shortness of breath, trembling, or fear of impending doom or death. A National Institutes of Health report states that moderate amounts of caffeine can trigger and magnify such panic attacks.

Pregnant women should note that several consumer advocate groups believe that caffeine is a teratogen, capable of causing cleft palate, heart abnormalities, missing digits, and other birth defects. Letters have been written to thousands of doctors and midwives urging that pregnant women be warned to avoid caffeine-containing drinks or OTC headache drugs. The FDA, however, states that their tests failed to demonstrate any conclusive evidence against caffeine as a teratogen. Just the same, the FDA has ruled that caffeine-containing products must be labeled to warn pregnant women and nursing mothers to avoid use. In another area, there is *some* evidence linking caffeine and xanthine intake to fibrocystic breast disease (noncancerous lumps in the breast).

Drug interactions: Caffeine combined with monoamine oxidase inhibitors such as Parnate and Nardil may result in a hypertensive crisis. Caffeine may increase the effects of thyroid drugs and amphetamines. Conversely, caffeine and sedatives are therapeutically incompatible—they nullify each other's effects. If an overdosage of Darvon (propoxyphene) is accidentally or intentionally taken, caffeine should not be given because of the possibility of fatal convulsions. Caffeine does *not* "sober up" persons who are under the influence of alcohol.

See also GUARANA

Cannabis

The term "cannabis" is used internationally to mean the flowering tops, leaves, and sometimes the stems and seeds of the hemp plant, *Cannabis sativa.* In American usage, marijuana means the same thing, but it must be understood that the potency of the plant will vary from nation to nation and even from state to state. A Mexican product (Acapulco gold) may differ in strength from a Hawaiian (Maui wowie) or from California-grown sinsemilla. North African or Indian cannabis, too, may have a unique potency and may be prepared in a special way. For further discussion, see the sections on hashish and marijuana.

Carbon Tetrachloride. *See* SOLVENTS AND INHALANTS

Carcinogen

If a substance is capable of inducing cancer, it is termed a carcinogen. Carcinogens occur in nature and as the result of chemical change or synthesis. The tars in cigarette and marijuana smoke contain large molecules called polycyclic hydrocarbons, and these have been shown to be carcinogenic. It appears that incomplete combustion of any organic substance (tobacco, charcoal, foods, fuels) can give rise to carcinogenic polycyclic hydrocarbons.

Unfortunately, many of the substances created by scientists in the laboratory have turned out to be carcinogens, as determined by tests in rodents and other laboratory animals. Critics hurry to point out that rodents are far removed from humans and that it isn't correct to extrapolate such test results to the human case. However, we cannot carry out tests for carcinogenicity in humans, and we do know that every chemical that causes cancer in humans also causes cancer in rodents, and thus the scientific community is generally convinced of the correctness of our present system of identifying cancer-causing agents.

Some of the old, familiar solvents such as chloroform, carbon tetrachloride, and benzene that we have long used and relied upon are considered now to be carcinogens. The careful home-owner and laboratory worker will check labels and consult with OSHA if there is any doubt about a substance in personal use.

Radiation (X rays, gamma rays) can induce cancerous growth. Avoid any unnecessary X rays. Insist that your dentist protect your body when he or she X-rays your teeth.

Cocarcinogens are agents that by themselves do not cause cancer but that when combined with another agent promote cancer formation. A famous example is alcohol combined with cigarette smoke; this combination is especially hazardous and is suspected of causing many a mouth, pharynx, larynx, and bronchial cancer.

Carter's Little Pills

Other name of active ingredient: bisacodyl
Source: synthesis
Pharmacology: contact-type, stimulant-irritant laxative
Doses: adults, 1 to 3 pills at bedtime; children over 3 years, 1 pill at bedtime
Bisacodyl, the active ingredient in this laxative, is related chemically to phenolphthalein (used in Ex-Lax). Both chemicals are stimulant-irritants to the large intestine, causing an increase in peristalsis and faster evacuation. However, it is generally agreed that stimulant laxatives are the least desirable because they can produce undesirable and sometimes dangerous side effects. And these adverse effects become more acute as users tend to rely more heavily on the stimulant laxative.

Although the manufacturers of this product recommend its use in children over 3 years of age, it is clearly unwise to do so, for two reasons. First, a young child's intestines should not be subjected to a powerful stimulant-irritant laxative. Second, to lead a child to laxatives at a young age is teaching the child to rely on unnatural stimulation for what should be a natural act. It is grievous to imagine a child of 6 or 7 getting accustomed to taking laxatives, and then relying on them for the next 60 to 70 years.

Carter's Little Pills are enteric-coated. That means they are designed to dissolve in the alkaline intestines and not in the acidic stomach, and therefore they must not be chewed. If you cannot swallow whole pills, do not attempt to use this product.

Misuse potential: high

Adverse effects: Powerful stimulants such as bisacodyl and phenolphthalein can empty the lower bowel completely, and it may take days for it to refill to the point where defecation is again normal. Anxious persons may feel that during this time they need more laxative, and if that doesn't work, even more. This has led many to a laxative dependence. Avoid becoming a slave to the laxative habit. Reject the unscrupulous ads that urge you to make a laxative a "member of the family." It is better to flush laxatives directly down the toilet without passing them first through your body.

Children under 3 years should not use this product. If you have nausea, vomiting, abdominal discomfort, or pain, do not use this product (using a laxative in impending appendicitis is very dangerous); avoid using this laxative within one hour of ingesting milk or an antacid.

Drug interactions: Some medications—such as ampicillin, tetracycline, and lincomycin—frequently cause loose, watery bowel movements. Combining a stimulant laxative with these drugs could result in a diarrhealike condition. Vitamin C and milk of magnesia also can cause diarrhea and should not be combined with a laxative. Paregoric (camphorated tincture of opium) is a constipating agent and would counteract the effect of a laxative.

See also DULCOLAX, LAXATIVES

China White

Illicit manufacture, distribution, sale, and use of heroinlike chemicals is big business, especially in underground laboratories on the West Coast. Chemists in some of these labs are quite sophisticated and can turn a few thousand dollars' worth of chemicals and equipment into illicit drugs eagerly sought after by upscale young professionals (and others) and worth literally millions of dollars.

Public, private, and governmental laboratories routinely receive samples of street drugs for analysis. These labs are our means of keeping current on what new (and old) narcotics, stimulants, and hallucinogens are on the American and world markets. In the past few years these labs have received a pure white powder sold on the street as "China White," ostensibly a synthetic heroin. Chemical analysis showed that it was not actually heroin but one of several other compounds. One report identified China White as alpha-methylfentanyl (or 3-methylfentanyl). Another identified it as MPTP (see the section on MPTP). Obviously there are no labeling requirements for street drugs, and it is impossible to prove the original nature of China White. Users are simply taking their chances on such street purchases.

There is a real danger in taking the so-called synthetic opiates like China White. Some of these drugs have been found to be extremely potent, while others are dangerously toxic. See the discussion of MPTP.

See also MPTP, FENTANYL, DESIGNER DRUGS

Chloral Hydrate

Other names: aquachloral suppositories, Noctec
Source: synthesis
Pharmacology: sleep-inducer (hypnotic)
Dose: Adult, hypnotic: 0.25–1 g taken 0.25–0.5 hour before bedtime or surgery. For sedation: 0.25 g 3 times a day. Do not exceed 2 g a day.

Chloral hydrate, a useful alternative to the barbiturates for inducing sleep, has had a long and colorful history. First synthesized in 1896, it is considered to be an effective sedative and hypnotic that is unlikely to induce tolerance, although it may be habit-forming. It disturbs REM sleep less than the barbiturates but does show some drug interactions. Chloral hydrate in combination with ethyl alcohol constituted the infamous "Mickey Finn" knockout drops. Although the potency of the preparation probably was overrated, chloral hydrate and alcohol offer a synergistic combination of CNS depressants that make sleep hard to resist. The knockout scam is still being played, but hookers today spike their victims' drinks with Ativan, scopolamine, or diazepam.

The half-life of chloral hydrate is short. It is metabolized in the liver to trichloroethanol, the active metabolite. Chloral hydrate is a Schedule IV drug under the 1970 Controlled Substances Act (see controlled substances) but is not currently a street drug of significant abuse. Since it can upset the stomach, it should be taken with a full glass of water.

Abuse potential: low

Adverse effects: Within 2 weeks of taking larger than usual therapeutic doses of chloral hydrate, tolerance and psychic dependence can develop. Chloral hydrate addicts who take heavy doses may develop physical dependence, with a withdrawal syndrome that can be serious or fatal. The syndrome is not unlike that seen with barbiturate dependence.

Some users report allergic reactions to this drug, including skin rash, hives, dermatitis, and itching. Occasionally a user will become disoriented, incoherent, or paranoid. Nausea, vomiting, gas, and diarrhea are occasionally reported, with gastric irritation.

Drug interactions: Chloral hydrate can increase or interfere with the body's breakdown of concurrently administered drugs such as coumarin anticoagulants, cortisone-type drugs, and several other types of drugs. Monoamine oxidase inhibitor drugs increase the sedative action of chloral hydrate. Taking an antihistamine drug concurrently with chloral hydrate can cause oversedation (sleepiness and lethargy).

WARNING: Avoid the combination of chloral hydrate and alcohol. The two together can easily produce oversedation.

See also SLEEP AIDS

Cocaine

Other names: coke, snow, coca, crack, rock

Sources: The plant *Erythroxylon coca,* grown in Bolivia, Colombia, and Peru

Pharmacology: brain and spinal cord stimulant; local anesthetic; vasoconstrictor

Dose of abuse: 25–100 mg intranasally

Cocaine, an alkaloid obtained from a South American plant, is a powerful stimulant to the central nervous system and to the heart. It is also a potent local anesthetic with its own built-in vasoconstrictor action.

Cocaine in any form can produce a compelling type of dependence; it is a very rewarding drug. One hundred years ago, Freud himself described its effects: exhilaration, lasting euphoria, increase of self-control, greater capability for work, elimination of fatigue, and complete elimination of the need for food or sleep.

Modern users describe cocaine's effects as the "perfect illusion." They think they are more competent, smarter, sexier, vigilant, masterful, productive, and full of energy. Thus, they say, cocaine is ego food.

Cocaine is a central nervous system (CNS) stimulant. This means that it excites the brain and spinal cord. It accomplishes this by stimulating the release of and blocking the brain's reuptake of dopamine and norepinephrine, two chemicals called catecholamines that are naturally present in the CNS and that account for mental alertness and excitation. With more catecholamines present, the brain is stimulated, eventually to the point of euphoria. In the brain, dopamine transmits impulses to the "pleasure center." Hence cocaine, by increasing dopamine levels, induces pleasureful sensations.

How can we explain the hold that cocaine can have over an individual? How can it be that people who should know better—including physicians themselves—can lose everything they have and nearly destroy themselves in their involvement with this substance?

The answer lies in the seductive and intensely coercive nature of the drug. Cocaine is one of the most powerful pharmacological reinforcers known, inducing pleasureful, seldom-achieved ecstatic experiences. But despite this, cocaine is the most unsatisfying of all of the major drugs of abuse. It produces ecstasy but never satisfaction, and the user feels compelled to "enjoy" it over and over again. In the heavy user, stopping the drug is likely to produce a mental depression with accompanying paranoia. This can be so intolerable as to border on the suicidal. Hence the abstainer is forced to return to the drug. The occasional social user may escape cocaine's clutches, but in up to 20% of other users, tolerance, insatiable craving, and ultimately ruin can occur. Laboratory animals trained to push a lever to receive a dose of cocaine will push the lever over 12,000 times finally to receive their drug. They will work for cocaine in preference to food even though they are starving.

Until recently, cocaine was believed to cause only a psychological (psychic) dependence; tolerance and physical dependence were believed not to occur. Now, however, some experts believe that when very high plasma concentrations of the drug are achieved through mainlining or smoking free-base cocaine for weeks or months, tolerance and ultimately physical dependence develop. Heavy coke users report that they are physically sick (withdrawal syndrome) when they abruptly terminate their cocaine.

Cocaine has additional pharmacological actions that are mediated centrally. These include an increase in heart rate and blood pressure, and hyperthermia (elevated body temperature).

Cocaine has long appeared in illicit traffic as the water-soluble hydrochloride salt, and in this form was sniffed into the nose or injected intravenously. Recently, the free-base form of cocaine ("crack") has become available for smoking. Made in a process that utilizes baking soda, the water-insoluble free-base form is rocklike and can be broken into pieces. Sometimes ether is used in the process, but ether constitutes an acute hazard because of its high flammability and tendency to form explosive mixtures with air. Entire buildings have blown up and burned down because of ether explosions that occurred in the process of making free-base cocaine.

Crack can be placed into a plastic pipe, heated to a vapor, and inhaled. This is termed smoking, but actually nothing is combusted. Free-base cocaine is easier to heat to a vapor than cocaine hydrochloride; hence the popularity of free-basing. Also, smoking free-base cocaine gets a big dose of the drug to the brain quickly. Crack comes in small, ready-to-smoke pieces selling for as little as $5.00.

Through the action of plasma esterases and liver enzymes, cocaine is rapidly metabolized in the body, and its effects usually wear off within an hour. But depending upon the dose, cocaine can show some effects for up to 5 hours, and it has appeared in blood samples for up to 10 hours following the last dose. Some users take it 4 to 12 times daily. Cocaine is typically flushed out of the urine in 24 hours, but its major metabolite (breakdown product) can be detected in the urine for up to 4 days after the last dose.

The military, the International Olympic Committee, sports teams, and many employers now routinely screen urine samples for the presence of cocaine. Benzoylecgonine, the major metabolite of cocaine, can be detected in the urine for 3 or possibly 4 days after last use, using thin-layer chromatography, or immunoassays such as EMIT or RIA (Abuscreen). If a urine sample shows positive on the screening test, a confirmatory test should be done.

The purity of cocaine street samples is a factor in possible overdosage. Some studies have shown that the average purity of street samples of cocaine hydrochloride varies from 13% to 75%, with most at about 48%. Drug Enforcement Administration data peg the average purity much lower, at about 13%. Free-base cocaine preparations such as crack usually are in the 90% range. A five-year study of street drugs by the Do It Now Foundation showed that only 45% of street cocaine samples were authentic; the rest contained adulterants or no cocaine at all.

Look-alike cocaine products have been promoted for years as "incense" or under such names as Toot, CocoSnow, Pseudo-Caine, SuperCaine, and Co-co kaine. Until recently, at least, they were legal, for although they looked like the real drug, they contained only nonprescription, over-the-counter-salable substances such as caffeine, phenylpropanolamine (PPA), or benzocaine. Many states have now passed laws specifying prison terms and fines for the possession, manufacture, advertising, or distribution of cocaine look-alikes.

If you need help with a cocaine problem, you can call a cocaine hotline, 800-262-2463 (or 800-cocaine). This number averaged 1200 calls a day in a recent year.

Abuse potential: high

Adverse effects: The cocaine user feels compelled to "enjoy" cocaine again and again. In the heavy user, this means tolerance and an ever-increasing dose until finally signs of toxicity appear. Convulsions and respiratory failure are possible, as is cardiovascular collapse or liver damage. The heavy user may hallucinate about the presence of insects ("snow bugs") on the skin. Violent behavior has been observed. Perforated nasal septa are seen in chronic snorters. Irritability, weight loss, and poor nutrition are characteristic of cocainism.

However, the most malignant aspect of heavy cocaine involvement is postuse depression and paranoia. The high is so euphoric and the mental depression that follows withdrawal is so intolerable (suicidal in depth) that the user is forced to return to the drug. For some people its use can only lead to more use, to insatiable craving, and ultimately to ruin. Four stages in cocaine's road to ruin have been described: Euphoria → dysphoria → paranoia → schizopsychosis.

At high risk of heavy cocaine use are strong, ambitious, competitive, well-educated individuals who strive for perfection and who are economically successful. They are intolerant of weakness or frailty in themselves or in others.

The acute toxicity of cocaine is becoming better understood, and there is now evidence that cocaine can affect the heart in a life-threatening manner. From admittedly limited studies, researchers have concluded that cocaine can cause sudden cardiac death, heart attack, irregular heartbeat, and heart muscle tissue damage. Cocaine causes the heart to beat rapidly and forcefully, but at the same time it can constrict vessels bringing blood to the heart. This can lead to fibrillation, in which the heart stops pumping effectively and quivers like Jell-O. Animal tests at the National Institutes of Health appear to show that the anesthetic effect of cocaine can sensitize the brain to later potentially fatal seizure attacks from small doses of the drug. In other words, using coke over a period of time can have a "kindling" effect that may mislead users into thinking they are taking a safe dose when in fact they are gradually lowering their brain's threshold for seizure and sudden death.

Drug interactions: Any stimulant drug, including amphetamines, epinephrine, dopamine, caffeine, or any monoamine oxidase inhibitor such as Parnate or Nardil, when combined with cocaine, can produce a critical overstimulation of the brain and cardiovascular system.

Codeine

Other name: codeine phosphate
Sources: the opium poppy, methylation of morphine
Pharmacology: narcotic analgesic, antitussive
Dose: 10–120 mg (tablets typically contain 15-, 30-, or 60-mg doses)

Codeine and morphine are alkaloids that occur in the opium poppy plant. Codeine makes up approximately 0.5% of the dried weight of opium and is very similar in chemical structure to morphine, from which most of it is prepared. Codeine is a narcotic analgesic; it occupies the same receptors in the brain as all of the opiates and therefore is capable of inducing tolerance and physical dependence. Codeine is a Schedule II drug under the 1970 Controlled Substances Act (see the section on controlled substances).

For 150 years codeine has been used as a pain reliever and antitussive (cough suppressant) and has earned the reputation of being a safe narcotic. As a pain reliever codeine is only about one twelfth as effective as morphine when given subcutaneously, but the ratio is more favorable when given orally. Codeine works best in combination with aspirin or acetaminophen, drugs that increase its painkilling activity. Thus we see prescriptions for aspirin with codeine, Tylenol with codeine, or Empirin or Ascriptin with codeine. Unfortunately, one serious adverse effect with codeine is nausea and vomiting.

Codeine suppresses coughs by depressing the cough reflex center in the brain. A 15-mg dose of codeine, while having no effect on pain, can control an irritating cough. Terpin Hydrate and Codeine Elixir is an exempt narcotic in some states (less than 15 mg of codeine per fluid ounce) and can be purchased without a prescription, a fact duly noted by some heroin addicts. Codeine is not considered to be as addicting a drug as morphine or heroin, but addicts can use it to maintain their dependency. Of course, there are other effective antitussives besides codeine. See the discussion of dextromethorphan in the section on cough remedies.

Abuse potential: medium. Codeine has less abuse potential than morphine and far less than heroin. When injected, codeine does not produce the euphoric "rush" seen in heroin use. For pain relief, codeine is often given by mouth, and the oral route does not lend itself to addiction liability the way heroin and morphine do. Nonetheless, codeine is abused; it will satisfy the craving for opiates.

Adverse effects: When codeine is used for pain relief, its most serious adverse effects are nausea and vomiting. Most users will experience this. Taking the drug with food will decrease the nausea; if you still have the problem, ask your doctor if you can reduce the dose or take the drug less often. Severe constipation can also result from the drug. Serious overdosage with codeine is likely to cause the person to fall asleep or become stuporous. The breathing rate may be seriously depressed and the pupils pinpoint in size. These adverse effects are about the same for any opium derivative, so it probably will do you little good to ask your doctor to switch to another. Driving an automobile under the influence of a narcotic depressant such as codeine can be hazardous.

Drug interactions: Codeine enhances the effects of all central nervous system drugs, other narcotics, tranquilizers, and sleep inducers; in some cases, extreme sedation or coma can occur. Monoamine oxidase inhibitors such as Parnate and Nardil increase the sedative action of codeine, but aspirin increases its painkilling action.

See also COUGH REMEDIES, MORPHINE, OPIATES

Colace. *See* LAXATIVES

Cold Remedies

The common cold has been judged the most costly single illness in the United States. More time is lost from work and school because of the common cold than because of all other diseases combined.

Most of the head colds we catch are caused by a virus. There is no known cure for this type of viral infection. All we can do is treat the symptoms and give the body time to manufacture interferon, which eventually helps overcome the viral infection.

The status of vitamin C (ascorbic acid) in head cold treatment or prevention is still unsettled. There is no doubt that vitamin C helps maintain the integrity of the mucous membrane and therefore is a prerequisite to good health. The difference of opinion lies in *how much* ascorbic acid we should ingest, and if colds can be prevented or ameliorated by this vitamin. Nobel laureate Linus Pauling, a prominent advocate of the merits of vitamin C, suggests daily doses in many thousands of milligrams. The federal government publishes an adult minimum daily requirement (MDR) for vitamin C of 30 mg and a recommended dietary allowance (RDA) of 45 mg. However much you decide to take, you should take it daily, for this water-soluble vitamin is not stored well in body tissues, and the body is not capable of synthesizing it. See the section on vitamin C for more discussion.

The sufferer from an acute head cold wants relief from a stuffed-up or runny nose (rhinitis), sneezing, or possibly a sore throat, headache, cough, or laryngitis. The following table lists ingredients in OTC cold products that are advertised to relieve these conditions. CAUTION: There is no evidence that antihistamines can prevent or cure the common cold; there is little or no scientific rationale for the use of an expectorant.

Of all the drugs in this table, the most potent are the decongestants such as phenylpropanolamine and pseudoephedrine. Some are discussed in their own sections in this book, but we can state here that these decongestants are sympathomimetics, patterned after the catecholamines, and are therefore potent medications. Besides shrinking nasal membranes and blood vessels, they can excite the CNS and stimulate the heart and circulatory system. Although it is true that their central actions are minimal, these side effects still exist to some degree, and the sensitive user may discover his or her heart beating at a faster rate after using them. In addition, some users of nasal decongestants experience a rebound congestive effect—their nasal congestion is even worse after the drug's effects wear off. This necessitates another dose of decongestant, and another, until the patient is sniffing all day long with no real relief. This can lead to a type of dependence that is difficult to correct. We reach the conclusion that since decongestants work only briefly and can have serious side effects, it is better to avoid them in the first place.

The FDA deplores the "shotgun" formulation of many cold

Drug Category	Condition Intended to Relieve	Examples of Drugs	Possible Adverse Effects
antihistamine	rhinitis	diphenhydramine, doxylamine, chlorpheniramine, pyrilamine	drowsiness
decongestant	stuffed-up nose or sinuses	oxymetazoline, phenylpropanolamine, pseudoephedrine, phenylephrine	increased blood pressure; excessive heart stimulation, insomnia
expectorant	accumulated sputum	ammonium chloride, guaifenesin, Terpin Hydrate	—
cough suppressant (antitussive)	persistent, unproductive cough	dextromethorphan, codeine phosphate, noscapine	drowsiness, stomach upset
analgesic-antipyretic	body aches, fever	aspirin, acetaminophen salicylamide	see sections on aspirin and acetaminophen

remedies: an antihistamine, a vasoconstrictor decongestant, aspirin (or acetaminophen), caffeine, and possibly vitamin C or a belladonna alkaloid. Thus to get one drug that might relieve a symptom, the user is forced to ingest four or five others that aren't needed, that are expensive, and that might have side effects or allergic potential. In addition, the advertising for many cold remedies is deplorable. Almost all contain the same ingredients, or at least very similar-acting drugs. So beware of the catchy ads that offer an "advanced formula, new strength, multisymptom, triacting, nighttime, daytime, great grape taste, maximum strength, maximum relief, vapor action, lemony flavor, new head and chest combination." It makes more sense to avoid the combinations and buy drugs individually, as needed, to avoid possible adverse effects of unnecessary medication. Note also that almost all the cold remedies we are discussing here can be bought generically at much less cost.

In summary, there is nothing you can take to cure a cold or even hasten recovery significantly. The OTC remedies that are heavily advertised are often shotgun products with clear-cut disadvantages to their use. If aching and fever accompany a cold, generic aspirin may be the drug of choice.

See also ANTIHISTAMINES, ASPIRIN, NYQUIL, PHENYL-PROPANOLAMINE, PSEUDOEPHEDRINE, SINUS PRODUCTS

Contac

Other names of active ingredients: phenylpropanolamine, chlorpheniramine

Source: synthesis

Pharmacology: decongestant, antihistamine

Dose: One caplet (containing 50 mg of phenylpropanolamine and 8 mg of chlorpheniramine) every 12 hours. Children under 12 years should use only as directed by a physician. If you have a high fever or if symptoms continue for more than 7 days, throw this product away and see a physician.

Heavily advertised for cold relief, this over-the-counter product contains the decongestant phenylpropanolamine and the antihistamine chlorpheniramine in a time-release capsule. In its actions, phenylpropanolamine is related to adrenaline and thus is able to cause constriction of blood vessels, an action that is the basis for its use as a decongestant. It works better when applied topically than when taken orally. No matter how taken, phenyl-propanolamine gets into the bloodstream and exerts its effect on the brain, heart, and blood pressure. Although this is of minimal consequence to most users, others may find their heart beating faster or their mind stimulated at bedtime after using Contac. Those who are most at risk are heart patients, hypertensives, hyperthyroid patients, digitalis users, glaucoma patients, and those who have difficulty emptying their urinary bladder. By the way, phenylpropanolamine is the same drug that is often used as an appetite suppressant, attesting to its brain-stimulating power.

Chlorpheniramine is an antihistamine. There is no evidence that antihistamines prevent head colds or even hasten recovery. They do have the adverse effect of making some users drowsy. Be careful about operating a car or complex machinery while under the influence of an antihistamine. What is more, the around-the-clock action of these time-release capsules means that you are under the influence of chlorpheniramine all day long.

Contac is very expensive. One store is selling this product for $5.17 for 20 caplets, or about $25 per hundred! If you wish, you may purchase the same ingredients individually and singly as generic drugs. The savings will be enough to cut the cost just about in half.

Misuse potential: medium

Adverse effects: Some users of Contac (especially children) may experience dizziness, insomnia, or nervousness (because of the stimulant decongestant). Contac possibly can make the following conditions worse: high blood pressure, diabetes, asthma, glaucoma, thyroid disease, and difficulty in urination due to enlarged prostate. Some users of Contact may experience inattentiveness while operating a vehicle or complex machinery.

Drug interactions: Do not combine this drug with alcohol, as too much sedation could occur. Do not take Contac if you are taking a drug for high blood pressure without first consulting your physician. Combining a monoamine oxidase inhibitor such as Parnate or Nardil with Contac could possibly result in dangerously high blood pressure. See your physician if you anticipate such a drug combination.

See also ANTIHISTAMINES, COLD REMEDIES, GENERIC DRUGS, PHENYLPROPANOLAMINE

Controlled Substances

The Federal Controlled Substances Act of 1970 regulates the use and distribution of thousands of drugs and chemicals available in the United States that have a high potential for abuse or dependence. Abuse of a drug means use or excessive use purely for pleasure, excitement, diversion, to get "high," to get "down," to be "cool," because of dependency, or use for a condition for which the drug is not medically indicated. These controlled substances fall into 1 of 5 possible schedules, depending on their potential for abuse. Schedule I lists drugs and chemicals that have high abuse potential and no current medical use. Schedule II identifies drugs that have a high potential for abuse but are used medicinally. The other three schedules list drugs in decreasing order as threats to society. The federal act (and similar state acts) specify fines and/or jail sentences for illegal possession or sale of controlled substances.

Examples of Schedule I drugs are para-fluorofentanyl, heroin, LSD, mescaline, tetrahydrocannabinol, peyote, and psilocybin. Examples of Schedule II drugs are benzedrine, Ritalin, Percodan, cocaine, codeine, morphine, methamphetamine, Demerol, Seconal, and Dexedrine. Lomotil is a Schedule V drug. Many thousands of drugs are not controlled because they pose little or no potential for abuse. Examples are aspirin, acetaminophen, laxatives, antacids, and antihistamines.

State laws for controlled substances are generally similar to the federal law, but the federal law would apply only to a product that has crossed a state line (been in interstate commerce).

The most severe penalty for breaking the federal law is a $50,000 fine and up to 30 years in prison. This type of punishment is reserved for those repeat offenders who intend to distribute large quantities of controlled substances.

Copper Bracelet

Other name: none
Source: mineral
Pharmacology: purported arthritis cure or treatment
Dose: worn on the arm or leg
The copper bracelet scheme is one of the most popular and

recurrent forms of arthritis rip-off. The advertisements for copper (or stainless steel) bracelets are among the most blatant examples of misrepresentation. One bracelet sold for $100, and the user was instructed to wear one of them on the left wrist and the other on the right ankle! Another ad warned that your old bracelet was becoming obsolete and you needed a new one.

Metallic copper is not absorbed through the skin and therefore can have no internal effect. Besides, arthritics don't need more copper. A scientific study showed that arthritics already have higher levels of copper in their bodies than do nonarthritics.

The copper bracelet "cure" has been refuted repeatedly by experts in court actions. The loss of money is not the least damage suffered by the purchaser, for the delay in seeking competent medical advice could result in progression of arthritic symptoms and a worsened condition for the patient.

See also QUACKERY

Coricidin

Other names of active ingredients: acetaminophen, Chlor-Trimeton (and in Coricidin D, phenylpropanolamine)

Source: compounding

Pharmacology: fever and pain reducer, antihistamine (and decongestant)

Dose: for adults and children 12 years and older, 2 tablets every 4 hours, not to exceed 12 tablets in 24 hours; for children 6–11, 1 tablet every 4 hours, not to exceed 5 tablets in 24 hours

Regular Coricidin contains Chlor-Trimeton (an antihistamine) and acetaminophen (a fever and pain reducer). Coricidin D adds a third drug, phenylpropanolamine (a decongestant sympathomimetic). Coricidin, sold as a cold and allergy product, is another example of a "shotgun" preparation. Like a blast of buckshot that probably will hit some target, shotgun drug combinations probably will relieve some symptom at the expense of much wasted therapeutic effort. The FDA has found a lack of evidence that these preparations work to cure colds or even hasten recovery. What is worse, if you have only a fever and take a shotgun drug, you are subjecting yourself to the possible adverse effects of the other, useless ingredients (see the section on phenylpropanolamine and the possible hazards in its use).

An alternative to products such as this one is to use only a drug for which there is a need. And you can purchase that drug singly and generically at a considerable savings.

Misuse potential: high

Adverse effects: Antihistamines can make one drowsy and reduce alertness when driving a car or operating machinery. Acetaminophen in the recommended dose probably will not cause significant adverse effects, but overdosing with acetaminophen can result in liver damage. Persons with a known history of liver disease should consult their physician before using acetaminophen. The phenylpropanolamine in Coricidin D (the same stimulant that is used as an appetite suppressant) can cause mental excitement and a rapid heart rate in sensitive people. If you have high blood pressure do not use Coricidin D without prior approval of your doctor.

Drug interactions: Combining alcohol with an antihistamine can cause one to become drowsy or overly sedated. Acetaminophen taken together with an oral anticoagulant can intensify the action of the anticoagulant and increase the chances of spontaneous bleeding. Combining acetaminophen with alcohol can increase the poisonous effects of both on the liver (avoid this combination, or see your doctor before using). The phenylpropanolamine in Coricidin D, when combined with epinephrine or other stimulants, can increase blood pressure, induce irregular heartbeat, or cause insomnia in susceptible users. The use of Parnate, Nardil, or any other monoamine oxidase inhibitor with phenylpropanolamine is strongly contraindicated.

See also ACETAMINOPHEN, ANTIHISTAMINES, COLD REMEDIES, PHENYLPROPANOLAMINE

Corn Removers

Corns and calluses are pretty much the same condition, but bunions and warts are unique foot problems. Pressure from tight-fitting shoes is the usual cause of corns, while friction or walking barefooted contributes to callus formation. In both corn and callus there is hyperplasia—abnormal increase in the horny layer of the skin—but in a callus there is no central core. Bunions are swellings of the bursae caused by various conditions, and warts are tumors of the skin caused most often by a viral infection.

The first goal in the treatment of corns and calluses is the elimination of the cause—that is, the source of the pressure or friction. However, the layperson also wants an OTC medicine that will remove the mass of tissue, and he or she turns to one of the products with supposed keratolytic activity. A keratolytic will dissolve or at least soften the keratin that makes up most of the horny layer of the skin.

Although there are many corn and callus remover products on the market with various ingredients, only *one* active ingredient does any good. This is the conclusion recently reached by a review panel of the FDA. The only corn and callus remover listed as safe and effective is salicylic acid. It can be applied in concentrations of 12–40% when used in pads, plasters, or discs, and in concentrations of 12–17% when used in liquids.

Here are the ingredients the FDA found to be *ineffective* in the treatment of corns and calluses: ascorbic and acetic acids, allantoin, belladonna, chlorobutanol, diperodone hydrochloride, ichthammol, iodine, methylbenzethonium chloride, methyl salicylate, and vitamin A.

Co-Tylenol

Other names of active ingredients: acetaminophen, chlorpheniramine, dextromethorphan, pseudoephedrine

Source: compounding

Pharmacology: pain and fever reducer, antihistamine, decongestant

Dose: 2 caplets every 6 hours, not to exceed 8 in 24 hours; for children 6–12 years, 1 caplet every 6 hours, not to exceed 4 in 24 hours for 5 days

This is another example of a "shotgun" preparation that, as pellets from a shotgun, is likely to hit something at the expense of much wasted effort. Co-Tylenol contains acetaminophen (pain and fever reducer), pseudoephedrine (nasal decongestant, sympathomimetic), chlorpheniramine (antihistamine), and dextromethorphan (cough suppressant). The FDA has long held that multicombination products such as Co-Tylenol lack evidence of safety and effectiveness. What would be worse, to obtain say fever relief with Co-Tylenol, one is subjecting oneself to the possible adverse effects of a potential sympathomimetic and two CNS depressants. Remember: There is no cure for the common cold, nor any drug that can even hasten recovery.

Co-Tylenol is quite expensive. One store is selling 50 doses for $8.69, or over $17 per 100. If one were to purchase each drug individually (as needed) and generically, the cost could be cut by half or more.

Misuse potential: high

Adverse effects: Antihistamines can make one drowsy and reduce alertness when driving a car or operating machinery. Acetaminophen in the recommended dose probably will not cause significant adverse effects, but overdosing with acetaminophen can cause liver damage. If you have a history of liver disease, consult your physician before using acetaminophen. Pseudoephedrine is a stimulant drug (also used as an appetite suppressant) that can cause restlessness, insomnia, and dryness of the mouth and throat in sensitive users. If you have high blood pressure, heart disease, or diabetes, consult your doctor before you use any pseudoephedrine product.

Drug interactions: Combining alcohol with acetaminophen can increase the poisonous effects of both on the liver. Avoid this combination, or see your doctor before using. Combining alcohol with an antihistamine can make one drowsy; watch this if you are to drive a car or operate machinery. Acetaminophen taken together with an oral anticoagulant can intensify the action of the anticoagulant and increase the chances of spontaneous bleeding. Pseudoephedrine, combined with epinephrine or any other stimulant, can increase blood pressure, cause irregular heartbeat, or induce insomnia in sensitive users. The use of Parnate, Nardil, or any other monoamine oxidase inhibitor with pseudoephedrine can result in dangerously high blood pressure (hypertensive crisis).

See also ACETAMINOPHEN, ANTIHISTAMINES, COLD REMEDIES, PSEUDOEPHEDRINE

Cough Remedies

The cough reflex is a highly desirable, protective mechanism initiated by the presence of mucus or a foreign irritant in the air passages. (In serious cases, a cough may have its origin in heart disease, bronchitis, or emphysema.) A cough is an explosive expulsion of air from the lungs to expel an obstruction, but if the cough reflex is triggered repeatedly without the irritant being removed, it becomes unproductive and possibly exasperating.

Treatment of such persistent cough consists of administering a drug that will suppress part of the network of nerves that make up the cough reflex arc. Actually, this suppression occurs in the so-called cough center of the brain, where the drug (termed an antitussive) makes nerve transmission through the center more difficult. In other words, it elevates the threshold for coughing. Usually the coughing isn't stopped, but it is reduced in frequency.

The two important antitussive drugs in use today are codeine and dextromethorphan. In some states it is still possible to buy Terpin Hydrate and Codeine Elixir without a prescription (in California, all codeine sales are restricted to prescription only). A 15-mg dose of codeine, corresponding to 1½ teaspoonfuls of Terpin Hydrate and Codeine Elixir, while having no effect on pain, can effectively suppress the cough center and control an irritating cough; this fact has made codeine a very popular antitussive drug. Unfortunately, codeine's narcotic actions make it an attractive alternative when heroin or morphine is unavailable, and some addicts will make the rounds of pharmacies, buying up all of the exempt Terpin Hydrate and Codeine Elixir they can find.

Dextromethorphan is a synthetic antitussive having no narcotic action or addiction liability. In 15- to 30-mg doses (1–2 teaspoonfuls of the typical syrup) it acts to suppress the brain's cough center. It can be purchased OTC in syrups and lozenges under many trade names; check the label to make sure. Dextromethorphan has become a very popular drug in place of codeine for treating coughs.

As a point of interest, heroin is an excellent antitussive, an action noted when heroin was first introduced (legally, then) into medicine in Germany in the 1890s.

As with all OTC preparations, it is important to read the label for the list of ingredients in the cough product you are about to purchase. Three well-known cough remedies contain 25% by volume of alcohol—50 proof. Others contain up to 20% alcohol. Some products contain large amounts of sugar, or antihistamines that can make one drowsy.

An expectorant is a drug that acts to loosen thick mucus, sometimes called phlegm, associated with a chest cold, and causes the mucus to be propelled upward in the bronchial tree so that coughing can remove it entirely. Tiny hairlike projections called cilia line the air passages, and it is through their wavelike motions that the phlegm is propelled upward. For smokers, a word of admonition: Cigarette smoke damages the cilia, rendering them incapable of normal functioning.

The problem with discussing expectorants is that there is little scientific evidence that they actually work. Terpin Hydrate and ammonium chloride, for example, are widely used, but their merits as expectorants lie more in tradition and long use than in scientific proof. Guaifenesin is included in many OTC products, but the FDA has little good to say about it. Potassium iodide appears to work in bronchitis or asthma, but it has gastric irritant adverse effects.

A persistent cough is a warning that something is wrong. It's better to get medical advice than to try to suppress the cough for an extended time.

See also CODEINE, COLD REMEDIES

Counterirritants

A counterirritant is a preparation that is applied locally to produce a mild, superficial irritation that is intended to relieve some other irritation or discomfort. Supposedly the counterirritation takes your mind off the original problem, or as the makers of Ben-Gay explain, the counterirritants "stimulate sensory receptors, including receptors of warm and cold. This produces a counterirritant response which alleviates the more severe pain. . . ." The relief is only expected to be transient and temporary. Methyl salicylate is the most widely used counterirritant.

The problems with these preparations are their lack of significant, prolonged pain relief and their relatively high cost. Aspirin or acetaminophen by mouth, or heat treatment probably would be far more effective and certainly less expensive. Then there are the unusual (weird?) ingredients added apparently to create customer appeal but not to accomplish any real relief. Absorbine Jr. contains wormwood; Heet contains capsicum, a powerful skin irritant. Many contain menthol, which smells nice but doesn't do much. Repeat users of counterirritants apparently believe that if it smells really strong or different and contains strange ingredients, it has to work. (See the section on placebos.) Vaporub contains oil of turpentine. Many accidental poisonings occur by ingestion of excessive amounts of oil of turpentine. The following table lists some popular counterirritants.

OTC Product	Ingredients	Rated Safe and Effective by the FDA?
Absorbine Jr.	wormwood, menthol, thymol	no
Aspercreme	triethanolamine salicylate (trolamine)	no
Ben Gay	methyl salicylate, menthol	yes
Icy Hot Balm	methyl salicylate, menthol	yes
Metholatum	methyl salicylate, menthol	yes
Myoflex	triethanolamine salicylate (trolamine)	no
Vaporub	menthol, camphor, eucalyptus oil, spirit of turpentine	no

Methyl salicylate (oil of wintergreen), found in many counterirritant products, is closely related to aspirin; if you have an aspirin or salicylate allergy, avoid such products. There have been reports of persons rubbing salicylate-containing counterirritant products over large portions of their body with consequent absorption of large amounts of salicylate into their bloodstream. This can produce salicylate poisoning, especially in children. The poisoning is characterized by mental excitation, fever, rapid breathing, ringing in the ears, difficulty in hearing, headache, dizziness, mental confusion, nausea, vomiting, and diarrhea.

See also SALICYLATES

Crack. *See* COCAINE

Crank. *See* METHAMPHETAMINE

Crystal. *See* METHAMPHETAMINE

D

Dalmane

Other name: flurazepam
Source: synthesis
Pharmacology: benzodiazepine-type minor tranquilizer, sleep inducer
Dose: 15–30 mg before retiring; in the aged or debilitated patient, the maximum initial dose should not exceed 15 mg. Dalmane comes in 15-mg orange-and-ivory capsules and in 30-mg red-and-ivory capsules.

Dalmane, along with Valium, Librium, Serax, and Halcion, is a benzodiazepine-type minor tranquilizer. Although the primary therapeutic use of minor tranquilizers is in the treatment of anxieties, fears, phobias, and other neuroses, Dalmane is promoted primarily as a hypnotic agent for the treatment of insomnia. It's one of our most heavily prescribed drugs, being in the top 24 nationwide.

Misuse potential: high
Adverse effects: Dalmane has a half-life of 24–72 hours, which means that a full day after your last dose you may still be under its brain-depressant effects. Driving a car or engaging in a hazardous occupation with a little Dalmane in your bloodstream could be risky, a conclusion supported by simulated and actual driving tests.

Since a physical addiction or a psychological dependence to Dalmane (indeed, to all benzodiazepine-type minor tranquilizers) can develop, especially after high doses for several months, the insomniac should be cautioned to use this drug only sparingly and briefly, and only in the presence of a real need. Do not mix flurazepam and alcohol, either right after the dose of flurazepam or later in the day (remember the long half-life); the two drugs combine to overdepress the CNS.

CAUTION: Roche Laboratories, the makers of Dalmane, clearly state that since benzodiazepines may cause fetal damage, they should not be taken during pregnancy. People with pulmonary diseases, including emphysema, should consult their physician before using flurazepam or Dalmane.

Drug interactions: Combining Dalmane with alcohol, CNS-depressant drugs, or monoamine oxidase inhibitor drugs can cause oversedation. Benzodiazepine-type minor tranquilizers may increase the effects of coumarin-type anticoagulants. When anticonvulsant drugs are taken concurrently with Dalmane, there may be an increase in the frequency and severity of seizures.

See also BENZODIAZEPINES, SLEEP AIDS

Darvon

Other names: propoxyphene, Darvon-N, Darvocet-N
Source: synthesis
Pharmacology: analgesic for mild to moderate pain
Dose: 32–100 mg. The usual dose is 65 mg (2 pink 32-mg capsules or 1 pink 65-mg capsule) every 4 hours as needed for pain. If the patient has kidney or liver disease, the dose should be lessened.

This mild analgesic is chemically related to methadone and is generally similar in action to the opiate narcotics. Darvon is prescribed for mild to moderate pain and is marketed alone or in combination with aspirin or acetaminophen (for pain associated with fever). Propoxyphene is available generically.

Darvon only partially suppresses the withdrawal syndrome in opiate addicts. Although it can produce psychological dependence, administration by the IV route can increase its potential for producing physical dependence.

Abuse potential: medium
Adverse effects: The FDA in 1979 estimated that 1000 to 2000 deaths a year are associated with propoxyphene, either alone or in combination with other drugs; the majority appear to be suicides. Respiratory depression is the usual cause of death in propoxyphene overdosage. The FDA has ordered that warn-

ings about the risk of death appear on labels for all propoxyphene products and is trying to discourage physicians and consumers from unnecessary medical use of the drug.

WARNING: Suicidal and alcoholic patients should not be given propoxyphene, nor should patients taking tranquilizers or antidepressant drugs. The FDA has warned about the use of this drug during pregnancy, since neonates can experience withdrawal if their mothers abuse the drug during pregnancy. Use care while driving a car when under the influence of propoxyphene.

Drug interactions: Alcohol's brain-depressant effects are additive; you may find yourself groggy or falling asleep if you ingest this combination. Likewise, propoxyphene combined with sleeping pills, sedatives, and tranquilizers may result in overdepression. Aspirin, salicylates, and acetaminophen can increase the analgesic effects of Darvon; heavy smoking may decrease them.

Datura. *See* JIMSONWEED

DAWN

This acronym stands for Drug Abuse Warning Network, a federal program for collection of information about drugs that are used and abused in cities across the United States. Drawing upon hospital emergency rooms, coroners' offices, physicians, and other sources, DAWN prepares a list of over 270 drugs and the cities in which they are having an impact, as based upon emergency room mentions. Drugs that are monitored include amphetamine, cocaine, heroin, LSD, marijuana, methadone, methaqualone, PCP, pentazocine (Talwin), and propoxyphene (Darvon).

Here is a list of some cities that report high drug abuse based upon emergency room mentions per million population; after each city is listed the drug or drugs that have high local use: Boston (cocaine); Buffalo (PCP); Denver (LSD); Detroit (heroin); Miami (marijuana, methaqualone, propoxyphene); New Orleans (marijuana); New York (cocaine, heroin); Washington, D.C. (cocaine, heroin, marijuana, PCP).

DAWN data do not represent a scientific sampling, and rankings are not absolute. Nevertheless, the information is generally accurate and useful.

Decongestants. *See* COLD REMEDIES,
PHENYLPROPANOLAMINE, PSEUDOEPHEDRINE

Decriminalization

When a drug or a substance is decriminalized by federal, state, or local law, it is not made legal. Rather, the severe penalties for a still illegal substance are reduced or minimized. Furthermore, the illegality can now be punished as a misdemeanor rather than a felony. For a felony one can be arrested, convicted, and given a permanent criminal record. Under a misdemeanor one may simply be fined a nominal amount, much like getting a parking ticket.

Decriminalization of marijuana was a popular movement in the late 1970s, and a total of 11 states acted to decriminalize. Most of them specified 1 ounce (28.35 g) as the maximum quantity of pot that could be possessed for consideration as a misdemeanor. Since 1980 the movement toward liberalized marijuana laws has been blunted by parent groups and antipot organizations, and no additional state has voted to decriminalize.

See also MARIJUANA

Demerol

Other name: meperidine USP
Source: synthesis
Pharmacology: narcotic analgesic
Dose: Adults: 50–100 mg orally or by injection every 3–4 hours as needed for pain. Tablets come in 50- and 100-mg strengths.

Demerol is a widely used, effective narcotic analgesic (pain reliever) that was accidentally discovered in 1939 by researchers who thought they had prepared an atropinelike drug. Demerol, which is chemically unlike morphine, produces almost all of the important pharmacological effects of morphine: analgesia, sedation, euphoria, and respiratory depression (it does not cause pinpoint pupils). It is an addicting drug to which tolerance develops and which upon abrupt removal produces withdrawal symptoms. In the opiate addict it can substitute for heroin or morphine because it occupies the same receptors in the brain. The ready availability of Demerol in hospitals has resulted in some physicians and nurses becoming physically dependent on it.

As a painkiller, meperidine is only about 15% as potent as morphine and is given in comparatively large 50- to 100-mg doses.

Abuse potential: high

Adverse effects: The most expected adverse reactions to meperidine are lightheadedness, dizziness, nausea, vomiting, sweating, and sedation. If such effects occur in a person who is up and about, they may be alleviated if he or she lies down. The most serious adverse effect is depression of respiration, with possible accompanying shock and cardiac arrest. Other users report weakness, headache, tremor, transient hallucination, disorientation, and visual disturbances. Dry mouth, urinary retention, and constipation may be seen in some users. Allergic reactions to meperidine include skin rash, itching, and redness. In patients with kidney dysfunction or who are taking large doses, a breakdown product may accumulate, producing central nervous system excitation and seizures. People with other disorders, too, such as dementia, untreated hypothyroidism, head injuries, and multiple sclerosis, may be extra sensitive to the central nervous system–depressing effects of Demerol and other narcotic analgesics.

CAUTION: Meperidine is not as effective given by mouth as given by injection. Its action is strongly potentiated when given together with phenothiazines or many other tranquilizers, and its dose should be reduced accordingly.

Drug interactions: Tricyclic antidepressants like Elavil can enhance respiratory depression produced by meperidine. When Demerol is given to a person taking monoamine oxidase inhibitor drugs, a serious excitation reaction can occur, with sweating, rigidity, and high blood pressure (this effect, however, is variable). Patients receiving other narcotic analgesics should take Demerol only with great caution because profound sedation or coma could result. Solutions of Demerol and barbiturates are chemically incompatible.

See also NARCOTIC ANALGESICS

DES. *See* DIETHYLSTILBESTROL

Designer Drugs

When a legislature enacts a law controlling a certain drug—that is, controlling its manufacture, possession, or sale—the nature of the drug is specified. Its specific chemical structure is identified. Recognizing that, an entrepreneurial chemist in a clandestine laboratory can design a new chemical substance that differs chemically only slightly from the original drug (this is termed a synthetic analog). The new "designer drug" is not controlled under the law because its structure is different, albeit slightly. Pharmacologically, it acts almost identically to the original drug. Hence the chemist has gotten around the law; he can sell his designer drug with impunity—that is, until the legislature gets around to changing the law to include the designer drug.

Fentanyl is a narcotic analgesic used legitimately in surgery. Alpha-methylfentanyl was one of the first designer drugs to appear on the street; it is 200 times more potent than morphine but very dangerous to use. MPTP, discussed in its own section in this book, is a designer drug whose structure is almost identical to that of Demerol.

Lawmakers are now designing their laws to anticipate the designer drug approach, and in the future it will be more difficult to circumvent the legal system. The Justice Department has placed one of the famous designer drugs, para-fluorofentanyl, on Schedule I of the controlled substances list.

See also CONTROLLED SUBSTANCES, FENTANYL, MPTP

Desoxyn. *See* METHAMPHETAMINE

Desyrel

Other name: trazodone
Source: synthesis

Pharmacology: antidepressant, unrelated to tricyclics, MAO inhibitors, or other known types

Dose: 50 mg 3 times a day; dose may be increased but should not exceed 400 mg a day for outpatients. Both 50-mg and 150-mg tablets are available.

Desyrel is intended for use in depressed patients, whether in the hospital or an outpatient, with or without prominent anxiety. Its exact mechanism of action is unknown, except that it is not related to tricyclic or tetracyclic antidepressants or to monoamine oxidase inhibitors. There is some evidence that it acts by inhibiting serotonin. Persons who are candidates for this drug include those with loss of interest in normal activities, increased fatigability, loss of sexual desire, feelings of worthlessness, difficulty in concentration, and thoughts of suicide.

Abuse potential: low

Adverse reactions: Drowsiness, dizziness, nervousness, fatigue, headache, insomnia, dry mouth, blurred vision, nausea, vomiting, joint pain, low blood pressure, and decreased appetite are some of the adverse effects that are sometimes seen.

WARNING: A large number of male patients taking Desyrel have reported persistent abnormal erection of the penis without sexual desire. In some cases surgery was required to correct the priapism, and in some of these cases permanent impotence resulted. Male patients experiencing this phenomenon should immediately discontinue the drug and report to their physician.

Drug interactions: Trazodone can increase the effects of alcohol, barbiturates, and other CNS depressants. Elevations of plasma Dilantin and dioxin levels have also been reported.

Dexatrim

Other name of active ingredient: phenylpropanolamine (PPA)

Source: synthesis

Pharmacology: anorectic (appetite suppressant for weight control)

Dose: 1 capsule (50 mg regular, 75 mg extra-strength) at 10:00 A.M. with a full glass of water

This over-the-counter product, heavily advertised for weight control, contains a hefty dose of the brain stimulant phenylpropanolamine (PPA). This drug will put you into an artificially excited state, much the same as you would experience if you were angry or acutely stressed. Of course, you will not feel like eating in such a state, and you will lose weight. However, a continual state of artificial excitement is highly abnormal. You may notice that your heart is beating rapidly or that you have difficulty getting to sleep at night. If you already have high blood pressure or a heart condition, you may actually be risking an attack involving the cardiovascular system. Furthermore, most of the users of an anorectic discover that when they stop taking the drug they gain back all the weight they lost. For these reasons, the FDA is highly critical of stimulants in weight control. And you should be, too.

Misuse potential: high. Many people find the brain-stimulant effects of PPA quite satisfying, and they come to rely on them. They are encouraged to use the drug, especially in the high 75-mg strength. They may find it desirable to increase the dosage, or to use the drug for days or weeks at a time.

Adverse effects: Users of PPA have reported headache, nervousness, a fast heartbeat, palpitations, dizziness, and insomnia. It would be wise to have your blood pressure checked while using this drug. CAUTION: Do not give this drug to a child under 12 years. For those between 12 and 18 years or over 60 years, consult your physician before using this product. Do not use any PPA product if you have high blood pressure, heart disease, kidney or thyroid problems, or if you are pregnant, lactating, or being treated for depression.

Drug interactions: Do not combine this product with any nasal decongestant, since overstimulation of the cardiovascular system may occur. For the same reason, strictly avoid concurrent use of epinephrine-containing drugs. Combining PPA with a monoamine oxidase inhibitor drug such as Parnate or Nardil may result in dangerously high blood pressure. This product will counteract the effects of any high-blood-pressure-lowering drugs you may be taking.

See also APPETITE-SUPPRESSANT DRUGS

Dexedrine

Other names: dextroamphetamine sulfate USP, dexies
Source: synthesis

Pharmacology: CNS stimulant, appetite suppressant, narcolepsy treatment

Dose: Individualized in narcolepsy, but usually 5–60 mg per day in divided doses; children narcoleptics 3–5 years of age, 2.5 mg daily to start; children narcoleptics 6 years and older: 5 mg once or twice daily to start. Dexedrine is supplied in 5-, 10-, and 15-mg capsules, 5-mg tablets, and an elixir containing 5 mg per teaspoonful.

Dexedrine is one of the most widely used amphetamines. Designed chemically to be similar to adrenaline (epinephrine), the amphetamines have very similar sympathomimetic properties. They stimulate the central nervous system (CNS), elevate the mood, improve physical abilities, subdue fatigue, increase blood pressure and respiration rate, dilate the bronchi, constrict blood vessels in the extremities, constrict nasal mucous membranes, and depress the appetite. Dexedrine is known chiefly for its ability to excite the brain and spinal cord.

The manufacturers of Dexedrine state that its use is indicated in narcolepsy (sleep epilepsy), in childhood attention deficit disorder with hyperactivity (previously known as minimal brain dysfunction), and for short-term control of obesity. Dexedrine acts by increasing the release of norepinephrine, a synaptic neurotransmitter; this results in a state of artificial excitement in which the brain is stimulated and the appetite is depressed.

As regards obesity control, the FDA strongly discourages the use of amphetamines, and Wisconsin and Maryland have passed legislation that virtually bans the use of amphetamines for the treatment of obesity. Critics cite the abuse of amphetamines in "fat clinics," the possibility of the development of dependence, and the futility of relying on a chemical crutch when real progress comes from within.

Dexedrine is a Schedule II substance (see the section on controlled substances); stiff penalties can be imposed for illegal possession or sale.

Abuse potential: high

Adverse effects: Dexedrine, like all of the amphetamines, is a stimulant to the brain, heart, and spinal cord. Because it can increase blood pressure and stimulate the heart, it must be used with caution or not at all in patients with cardiovascular conditions. People who use Dexedrine typically develop a tolerance to it—that is, they must take ever larger and larger doses to get the same effect. Watch out for such development of tolerance, and stop taking the drug if you see it developing. If you have glaucoma or an overactive thyroid gland, take this drug only with the approval of your physician. Dexedrine can cause sleeplessness, irritability, and restlessness sufficient to interfere with ordinary daily functioning. It can cause dryness of the mouth, nausea, abdominal cramps, and diarrhea.

Drug interactions: WARNING: Strictly avoid concurrent use of Dexedrine with any monoamine oxidase inhibitor, since a dangerously high rise in blood pressure could result (hypertensive crisis). Dexedrine interferes with the antihigh-blood-pressure actions of Aldomet, Apresoline, and reserpine. Adrenergic blockers such as Inderal are also inhibited by Dexedrine. Concurrent use of any amphetamine with a tricyclic antidepressant such as Elavil could result in overstimulation of the brain. Lithium carbonate, taken at the same time as Dexedrine, can block the stimulatory effects of the former. If Dexedrine is given to a person who has overdosed on propoxyphene (Darvon), fatal convulsions can occur. Any amphetamine can counteract the sedative effects of antihistamines.

See also AMPHETAMINES, SYMPATHOMIMETICS, RITALIN

Diarrhea Products

There are many causes of diarrhea: bacterial or viral infection; drugs such as antibiotics, laxatives, or cathartics; and food intolerance. Chronic diarrhea may have its origin in gastrointestinal pathology or in psychological factors; it requires a physician's treatment.

Most of the prescription and OTC diarrhea products typically are directed against the symptoms of diarrhea. However, an FDA panel on antidiarrheal products concluded that almost all the OTC products on the market lacked evidence of either safety or effectiveness, the only exceptions being opiates (such as paregoric) and polycarbophil. Lacking evidence of effectiveness were the following purported antidiarrheal agents: alumina powder, attapulgite, belladonna alkaloids, bismuth salts, calcium carbonate, calcium hydroxide, sodium carboxymethylcellulose, charcoal, kaolin, lactobacilli species, pectin, salol, and zinc phenolsulfonate. Products containing variously these ineffective ingredients include Donnagel, Kaodene, Kaopectate, Pepto-Bismol, and Rheaban.

Opiates are effective antidiarrheals because the morphine in them shuts down peristalsis (intestinal motility). They are safe and effective in doses of 15–20 mg of opium or 1.5–2.0 mg of morphine (that's 1 teaspoonful of paregoric); at these low doses there is very little possibility of one becoming addicted. Another name for paregoric is camphorated tincture of opium. For more on paregoric, see its section in this book.

Present evidence points to the conclusion that you are wasting your money when you buy most of the antidiarrheal products on the market. Most (but not all) of the acute diarrheal attacks we experience are self-limiting and will clear up spontaneously without the use of any chemical agent. If high fever accompanies the diarrhea or if the diarrhea lasts for more than 2 days, consult a physician.

Diazepam. *See* VALIUM

Diethylstilbestrol

Other names: DES, former "morning after" pill
Source: synthesis
Pharmacology: synthetic nonsteroidal estrogen
Dose: 0.2–0.5 mg daily is usual, but dose should be individualized to smallest quantity that will be effective
CAUTION: DIETHYLSTILBESTROL SHOULD NOT BE USED AS A POSTCOITAL CONTRACEPTIVE. IT SHOULD NEVER BE USED FOR ANY PURPOSE DURING PREGNANCY.

In 1938, responding to the great demand for medicinal estrogen, chemists synthesized the first nonsteroidal estrogen, diethylstilbestrol, or DES. It was found to be highly potent and was widely used for, among other things, threatened abortion. Mothers of perhaps several million children were treated with DES in the 1940s. Many years later the discovery was made of an increased incidence of cervical and vaginal cancer in the daughters of women who took DES in their first trimester. The cancer typically shows up when the daughters are in their late teens or early twenties. In addition, noncancerous changes in the daughters' reproductive organs are common. For this reason DES should never be used for any purpose during pregnancy.

Later DES became popular as the "morning after" pill, given in large doses (25 mg) soon after sexual intercourse to prevent any fertilized ovum from implanting. There are other, better "morning after" pills now available (for example, prostaglandins), and the FDA now strongly discourages this use of DES and has withdrawn from the market the 25-mg tablets.

Today, Eli Lilly and Company markets DES for the treatment of vascular problems associated with the menopause, plus atrophic vaginitis, female hypogonadism, female castration, ovarian failure, and for certain cancers. Its use should be for brief periods in the lowest dose that will accomplish the results.

DES has long been used in cattle to promote growth and hasten arrival on the market. FDA regulations require termination of DES use long enough before slaughter so that no significant quantities of the chemical remain in the meat sold to the consumer. Just the same, critics decry this practice, and it is possible that the FDA will ultimately ban all use of DES in animals.

DES is an estrogen—albeit synthetic—and one can expect the side effects and adverse reactions typical of estrogenic drugs.

Misuse potential: high

Adverse effects: Diethylstilbestrol has many potentially serious effects on six different organs or systems of the body. There is a statistical relationship between the use of any estrogen and cancer of the lining of the uterus. In women with an intact uterus, diethylstilbestrol can cause breakthrough bleeding, candidiasis of the vagina, and symptoms resembling cystitis. With this drug there have been reports of breast tenderness, nausea, vomiting, abdominal cramps, discoloration of the skin, loss of hair, intolerance of contact lenses, dizziness, headache, mental depression, water retention, and reduced tolerance to carbohydrates.

CAUTION: DES—and estrogens generally—should not be used in persons with undiagnosed genital bleeding, a history of blood clot problems, a predisposition to gallbladder disease, elevated blood pressure, or a history of jaundice.

Drug interactions: Diethylstilbestrol and other estrogens increase the body's metabolism of calcium and phosphorus; this can cause problems in patients whose kidneys are working poorly. Taken concurrently, phenobarbital and other barbiturates increase the body's metabolism of estrogens. If a patient is on thyroid replacement therapy and takes an estrogen, he or she may have to increase the dose of thyroid drug.

See also ESTROGENS

Diet Pills. *See* APPETITE-SUPPRESSANT DRUGS

Di-Gel. *See* ANTACIDS

Dimethyl Sulfoxide

Other names: DMSO, $(CH_3)_2SO$
Source: derived from wood
Pharmacology: in humans, a treatment for cystitis (a bladder condition); in horses and dogs, a treatment to reduce swelling due to trauma
Dose: infused as a 50% solution

DMSO stands for dimethyl sulfoxide, $(CH_3)_2SO$, an industrial solvent derived from wood during paper production and used since the 1940s as a degreaser or cleaning solvent. In 1963 the University of Oregon Medical School reported that DMSO, when rubbed on the skin, showed remarkable penetrating power and was quickly absorbed into the body, where it relieved pain and inflammation. In a short time word spread about this "miracle" drug, and it soon became a "sure cure" for arthritis, sprains, burns, herpes infections, and high blood pressure.

Whether applied to the skin or taken internally, DMSO rapidly enters the bloodstream and soon appears on the breath with an unmistakable garliclike odor. When used topically (for example, in an ointment) it breaks down the skin's natural barrier to bacteria. Some people are severely allergic to DMSO.

The FDA has been looking at DMSO for many years but has

steadfastly refused to approve it for uses for which it has not been shown to be safe and effective. For example, the FDA says that DMSO's powerful penetrating action could cause an insecticide on a gardener's skin to be carried accidentally into his or her bloodstream. The FDA has approved DMSO for use in certain bladder conditions and as a veterinary medicine for topical use in nonbreeding dogs and horses. Meanwhile, the 99% industrial solvent solution continues to be sold at roadside stands and gas stations at exorbitant prices. It attracts a large following, and it is legal in Florida and Oregon. One DMSO advocate claims that the FDA is engaged in a "witch-hunt" against the drug. Little progress is being made on a final solution of the DMSO controversy.

Misuse potential: high

Adverse effects: The FDA is concerned about the facts that DMSO breaks down the skin's resistance to bacteria and that some people are highly allergic to it. Allergy is explained by the fact that DMSO causes the release of histamine. DMSO has been shown to cause opacity in the lenses of the eyes of dogs, but this has not been found to occur in humans. DMSO also can cause reddening of the skin, nausea, and the risk of blurred vision.

Drug interactions: Dimethyl sulfoxide can block the effectiveness of the antiarthritis drug sulindac.

Dimethyltryptamine

Other name: DMT
Source: plant, illicit synthesis
Pharmacology: hallucinogen
Dose: approximately 1 mg/kg, or about 70–80 mg for an adult male

Dimethyltryptamine, a hallucinogen that has a long history of use in South America, is obtained by illicit synthesis and is infrequently used in the United States. Chemically it is related to the amino acid tryptophan and the hallucinogens LSD and bufotenine; it appears on the street as a brown solid with an odor similar to that of mothballs. DMT is a federally controlled substance.

DMT is ineffective when swallowed, so it is usually inhaled in the smoke of a marijuana joint or cigarette to which it has been added. When it is inhaled or injected, the psychedelic effects begin almost immediately but last less than an hour. This is why it is sometimes called the businessman's lunch trip.

Frequent use of DMT causes rapid development of tolerance. Several drug-free days or a week of abstinence would be necessary before the drug would again produce hallucinations.

Abuse potential: high

Adverse effects: Any hallucinogen is potentially a dangerous drug because the possibility always exists that the user will experience highly unpleasant alterations in the perception of reality. Some users may feel that they are going out of their mind; a very few others may experience a psychotic breakdown. When 70–75-mg doses of DMT were given to normal subjects, they reported nausea, dizziness, tremor, increased heart rate, and elevated blood pressure.

Drug interactions: Concurrent use of other hallucinogens or mind stimulants such as epinephrine or amphetamines can result in acute overstimulation of the brain.

DMSO. *See* DIMETHYL SULFOXIDE

DMT. *See* DIMETHYLTRYPTAMINE

Doan's Pills

Other name for active ingredient: magnesium salicylate
Source: synthesis
Pharmacology: painkiller
Dose: for adults only, 2 tablets (325 mg each) with a full glass of water every 4 hours, not to exceed 12 pills in 24 hours

The active ingredient in Doan's Pills is magnesium salicylate, intended for relief of headache and occasional minor pain. Magnesium salicylate is a salt of salicylic acid, and like all of the other salicylates, including aspirin, it has analgesic properties. This product works to relieve headache, and the FDA has approved it as safe and effective for the use intended.

You should know, however, that aspirin is every bit as effective and can be purchased generically at much less cost. Further, the precautions against using aspirin in the last three months of pregnancy apply just as well to magnesium salicylate.

Misuse potential: low. However, if you plan to take this product for relief of arthritis, see your physician first. Magnesium salicylate can relieve arthritis, but if the dose is not adequate, only pain will be relieved and not the progression of the disease.

Adverse effects: Some people are powerfully allergic to salicylates; they must avoid this product. If you are pregnant, or have stomach ulcers, bleeding tendency, or gout, do not take this product unless you have discussed your condition with a physician. Because magnesium salicylate increases the amount of magnesium the kidneys have to eliminate, this product should not be used by persons with advanced kidney disease.

Drug interactions: Ammonium chloride and other drugs that acidify the urine should be given with caution to patients receiving salicylates since they can retard the elimination of the drug. Antacids, combined with high doses of salicylates, can alter serum levels of the latter. In persons receiving heparin, salicylates should be given with caution; the same appears to be true with indomethacin. Salicylates decrease the desired actions of probenecid (Benemid).

See also ASPIRIN, SALICYLATES

Donnagel

Advertised as an OTC treatment for diarrhea, Donnagel is one of the worst examples of a "shotgun" formulation. It contains kaolin, pectin, hyoscyamine, and atropine. The FDA has concluded that all these drugs lack evidence of safety or effectiveness. To make matters worse, these ingredients can cause serious adverse effects, including dryness of the mouth, blurring of vision, and difficulty in urination.

There is good reason to conclude that you are wasting your money and your trust on Donnagel as a means of relief of diarrhea.

See also DIARRHEA PRODUCTS

Dopamine

Other name: Intropin
Source: synthesis

Pharmacology: heart stimulant, shock treatment, increases kidney blood flow

Dose: variable; given by IV infusion

A close chemical relative of norepinephrine is dopamine (dihydroxyphenethylamine). This catecholamine is important primarily in the brain, but there are also receptors for it in the heart and kidneys. Dopamine is the neurotransmitter for (1) the brain's extrapyramidal system (coordination and integration of fine muscular movement, such as picking up small objects); (2) the brain's mesolimbic system (memory and emotions); and (3) the hypothalamic-pituitary axis (release of the hormone for lactation). In Parkinson's disease, the dopamine content of the caudate nucleus portion of the brain is found to be far below normal. Parkinsonism is treated by giving the patient L-dopa, the biogenetic precursor to dopamine (L-dopa readily passes the blood-brain barrier; dopamine does not).

Dopamine is excitatory to the brain. The antipsychotic major tranquilizers work by blocking dopamine receptors in the brain. Dopamine is available commercially as Intropin, a pressor agent used in the treatment of shock. It has the typical catecholamine action of increasing cardiac output and raising blood pressure. IV administration of Intropin has little effect on the CNS because the drug does not readily pass the blood-brain barrier.

Some researchers have proposed a dopamine hypothesis of mental illness. They believe that an excessive production of dopamine in the brain results in the signs of schizophrenia. Support for this theory is found in the fact that the major tranquilizers (the antipsychotics) work by blocking dopamine receptors in the brain.

Drug interactions: Combining dopamine with monoamine oxidase inhibitor drugs can cause dangerously high blood pressure. Cyclopropane or halogenated hydrocarbon anesthetics must be avoided when dopamine has been administered. Since both dopamine (in high doses) and the ergot alkaloids are powerful vasoconstrictors, combining them may cause dangerous peripheral constriction.

See also CATECHOLAMINES, ADRENERGIC, SYMPATHOMIMETIC, PARKINSON'S DISEASE

Doriden. *See* GLUTETHIMIDE

Downer

The term "downer" refers to any drug that causes a depression in the brain (or central nervous system). The barbiturates are the classical examples of downer drugs, but the term could be extended to other CNS depressants, such as the minor tranquilizers or even the antihistamines.

Nembutal, Amytal, and Seconal are examples of barbiturates that are street drugs of abuse. In doses of 50–100 mg or more these drugs will make the user feel woozy, carefree, or untroubled by reality. The user calls this getting "high" or "spaced out." Actually, the drug is depressing the brain and interfering with motor coordination skills needed for driving a car, operating machinery, or even lesser activities. As the dose of barbiturate is increased, the user can become acutely intoxicated, slurring his speech and staggering about, at high risk of having an accident.

Overdosing on a downer can be treated in several ways. In 3–6 hours the liver will metabolize most of the dose and the person will begin to come out of the depression. Alternatively, "upper" drugs can be given to counteract the depression. An upper is a brain-stimulant drug; probably the most readily available example is caffeine. However, one should not rely on caffeine to reverse the depression caused by an overdosage of a barbiturate. Rather, seek immediate medical attention.

Doxylamine

Other name: Decapryn
Source: synthesis
Pharmacology: antihistamine, sleep-inducer
Dose: 7.5–25 mg

This antihistamine, comparable in potency to diphenhydramine (Benadryl), is used in OTC products sold as sleep aids, cold medicines, and cough mixtures. It is contained in, for example, Contac, Formula 44, NyQuil, and Unisom in typical "shotgun" products (see the section on cold remedies). It also has been included in certain look-alike drugs to simulate the effects of "downer" drugs.

Antihistamines cannot cure the common cold or even hasten one's recovery, and if you are taking this drug as a cold remedy you are wasting your time. However, antihistamines are central nervous system depressants, and they can help some people get to sleep at night. If you must take something to get to sleep, you are better off with this drug than with a barbiturate. You may discover, however, that you still are a little groggy the next morning, and that is why the makers of doxylamine-containing products caution you not to drive a car or operate machinery if you are taking their drug.

Misuse potential: low

Adverse effects: Some people who take this drug will experience dryness of the mouth, dizziness, difficulty in urination, nausea, vomiting, and double vision.

Drug interactions: Concurrent use of any central nervous system depressant, such as alcohol, barbiturates, phenothiazines, or tranquilizers, with any antihistamine can result in dangerous sedation of the brain.

See also ANTIHISTAMINES, COLD REMEDIES, LOOK-ALIKES, SLEEP AIDS

Dristan

Other names of active ingredients: phenylephrine, acetaminophen, chlorpheniramine

Source: compounding

Pharmacology: decongestant, pain and fever reducer, antihistamine

Dose: adults, 2 tablets every 4 hours, not to exceed 12 tablets in 24 hours; children, 6–12 years, 1 tablet every 4 hours, not to exceed 6 tablets in 24 hours

Promoted for treatment of colds, flu, and sinusitis, Dristan is another example of a "shotgun" product that, like pellets from a shotgun, is likely to hit something at the expense of much wasted therapeutic effort. The phenylephrine in Dristan (5 mg per dose) has been used as a cardiovascular stimulant for raising blood pressure and is a potent drug. If you take Dristan for a runny nose, you can't escape getting a dose of phenylephrine. Remember also that no drug can cure the common cold or even hasten recovery from it. NOTE: The decongestant used in Dristan products can be either phenylpropanolamine, pseudoephedrine, phenylephrine, or oxymetazoline, depending on whether you are using the analgesic capsules or tablets, the nasal spray, or the nighttime liquid.

The FDA has long held that multidrug products such as this one lack evidence of safety and effectiveness. What is more, they are expensive. If you were to purchase each drug generically and individually (as needed), you could cut your costs in half.

Misuse potential: high

Adverse effects: Antihistamines can make one drowsy and reduce alertness when driving a car or operating machinery. Acetaminophen in the recommended dose probably will cause no significant adverse effects, but overdosing with acetaminophen can cause liver damage. If you have a history of liver disease, consult your physician before using this product. Phenylephrine is a stimulant to the heart and brain. If you suffer from heart disease, high blood pressure, diabetes, glaucoma, asthma, or have difficulty in urination, do not use this product without first consulting your doctor. Phenylephrine can cause insomnia in sensitive users.

Drug interactions: If you use alcohol while taking this product, you could become drowsy and at risk when driving a car or operating machinery. Combining alcohol with acetaminophen can increase the poisonous effects of both on the liver. Avoid this combination, or see your doctor before using. Phenylephrine combined with epinephrine or any other stimulant can dangerously increase blood pressure in sensitive users. The use of Parnate, Nardil, or any other monoamine oxidase inhibitor with phenylephrine can result in dangerously high blood pressure (hypertensive crisis).

See also ACETAMINOPHEN, ANTIHISTAMINES, COLD REMEDIES

Drug Allergies

There is no way to predict with certainty who will be allergic to drugs, or to which drugs a person might be allergic. However, you should be especially careful if you have a history of drug allergies or if you are asthmatic. Further, if you are in the high-risk category, you should be extra careful to avoid the following drugs or chemicals:

FD&C Yellow No. 5, also known as tartrazine, is a synthetic yellow dye approved for use in prescription drugs and foods; it can cause allergic reactions, including bronchial asthma in certain susceptible persons. Such sensitivity is frequently seen in patients who also have an aspirin allergy. Some drug manufacturers are removing FD&C Yellow No. 5 from their prescription products. Smith, Kline & French, for example, have removed it as the coloring agent in their Thorazine tablets. If you suspect that you are allergic to any dye, check with your pharmacist to determine if any coloring agent has been added to the drug prescribed for you.

Chemically, the name "sulfite" refers to salts of sulfurous acid such as the sodium salt Na_2SO_3. But in the area of allergic sulfite reactions, sodium sulfite is equivalent to sodium metabisulfite ($Na_2S_2O_5$), sulfur dioxide, and sodium bisulfite ($NaHSO_3$), all of which can produce severe reactions in sensitive people. For example, shortly after eating sulfite-sprayed or dipped produce at a restaurant, some people experience flushing, difficulty in breathing, hives, itching, and a fall in blood pressure. The allergic reaction can be severe, indeed, as shown by the 12 deaths recently attributed to sulfites. Sulfites are sometimes found in soft drinks, fruit juices, canned vegetables, frozen pizza, cake mixes, sausages, and pickled foods; most wines and some beers contain sulfites. If you are allergic, it's very important to read labels or ask questions. Asthmatics appear to be most at risk of reacting to sulfites; some 5–10% of them will show a sensitivity. However, about 30% of sulfite reactions have occurred in healthy persons with no history of allergies. The FDA has banned the use of sulfites in certain foods, but the sulfite-sensitive person must constantly be alert to accidental exposure.

See the section on aspirin for a discussion of its well-known ability to cause allergic reactions.

See also ADVERSE REACTIONS TO DRUGS

Drug Interactions

When a person takes two or more drugs at the same time, it is possible in some cases that one drug will have an effect upon the pharmacological action of the other. This effect may be either an enhancement or a reduction of activity—that is, one drug may heighten the action of another, or resist it. Enhancement may be the result of simple additive action, as when alcohol's CNS depressant effects are added to those of an antihistamine. Or the enhancement may result from a *synergistic* action—that is, a mutual potentiation that results in a superadditive effect. Synergism is like $2 + 2 = 5$. Ethyl alcohol and barbiturates are notoriously (and dangerously) synergistic, for they mutually potentiate depression of respiration. Aspirin can enhance the action of anticoagulants to the point of inducing hemorrhage.

Enhancement of drug action also can result if the body enzymes that usually catalyze its destruction are inactivated or inhibited by competition from another drug. Further, the serum level of a drug can be significantly raised if the drug is displaced from its binding sites by another drug.

An example of drug antagonism can be seen in chronic alcohol users who do not respond to Valium. This is because the alcohol has induced the formation of liver enzymes that cross over and also metabolize the Valium. Smokers may discover that they require extra-large and more frequent doses of a certain analgesic to get pain relief. This also is probably due to nicotine's stimulation of liver enzymes that catalyze the breakdown of an analgesic.

Physicians and pharmacists know of hundreds of combinations of interactive drugs, some of them life-threatening. It is best to consult your health professional when you are multimedicating. It is also wise to take only one drug at a time (if that is possible) and to limit your use of OTC drugs to those *really* necessary. Read the labels of OTC drugs. OTC antacids can seriously reduce the body's absorption of the antibiotic tetracycline.

Drugs can interact with food, too. Tetracycline antibiotics can lose their effects if taken with milk or dairy products. Monoamine oxidase inhibitors when combined with aged cheese, Chianti wine, pickled herring, fermented sausages, salami, pepperoni, yogurt, sour cream, livers, canned figs, or beer can produce a dangerous hypertensive crisis. Oral contraceptive drugs are known to lower blood levels of folic acid and vitamin B_6.

Drug Rip-offs

The purchase of any drug on the street is chancy at best and a complete rip-off at worst. According to Christine Dye, d.i.n. publications, Phoenix, Arizona, the street drugs that are most likely to be adulterated, misrepresented, diluted, or substituted are: amphetamines, heroin, mescaline, Quaalude, psilocybin, and cocaine (in that order). The deceit can run as high as 90%. These figures are from analyses made nationwide over a 5-year period.

What street drugs had the least deceit? MDA/MDM, LSD, and marijuana.

Drugs in Sports

The three types of drugs that have been used in sports training or competition are: CNS (psychomotor) stimulants, anabolic steroids, and painkillers. Examples of CNS stimulants that have been used are cocaine, amphetamines, caffeine, pemoline (Cylert), methylphenidate (Ritalin), and phenmetrazine (Preludin). Because these drugs excite the brain, increase heart rate and blood pressure, and stimulate physical exertion, they are likely to be used by athletes engaged in highly competitive, physically demanding contests. Their use can be dangerous because they add powerful external stimulants to those already being secreted by a stressed body.

Anabolic steroids are synthetic, hormonelike drugs that originally were prescribed for hospital patients who needed to increase their buildup of body protein tissue, as in anemia or postsurgical debilitation. (Anabolism is the use of body processes to grow tissue, build molecules, or increase actions that incorporate nitrogen into the body.) Later, athletes began taking anabolic steroids in the belief that they could build bigger bodies and gain a competitive edge. The practice is now open and widespread. Drugs used include Stanozolol, Nandrolone, Clostebol, Methenolone, and Oxymestrone. However, not all experts agree that the steroids actually build bigger muscles; many state that exercise in the accompanying training program produces the results.

All anabolic steroids are related chemically to the male sex hormones and can produce serious side effects in the user: testicular atrophy, impaired liver function, high blood pressure, and prostatic and liver cancer. Female users of anabolic steroids can experience menstrual irregularity, baldness, enlargement of the clitoris, and loss of body curves. Testosterone itself is being used in sports for its anabolic effects, as is growth hormone given by injection. There is no scientific evidence that growth hormone can improve athletic performance. The use of drugs to enhance physical performance is called doping. The International Olympic Committee (IOC) had defined doping as either the use of substances foreign to the body, or physiological substances in abnormal amounts, or drugs used by abnormal methods with the goal of obtaining unfair advantage during competition. The IOC now requires winners of events to submit a urine sample within 1 hour of competition to check for the presence of amphetamines, anabolic steroids, pain relievers such as codeine, and other drugs. Caffeine is permitted in the urine in concentrations up to 15 mcg per ml.

Although anabolic steroids are sold in the United States by prescription only, they are sold OTC, as much as you want, in Mexico. Smuggling these drugs into the United States is a federal offense.

Although most people agree that drugs have no place in sports, the practice continues widespread around the world.

See also AMPHETAMINES; ANABOLIC STEROIDS; STEROIDS; DRUGS, TESTING FOR

Drugs, Testing for

The presence of a drug in the human body can be demonstrated by examining urine, blood, and/or breath. Blood is the most valuable fluid, for what is in the urine or on the breath is only a reflection of what is in the blood. However, urine samples are the most convenient to collect and store.

Today Olympic committees, employers, law enforcement agencies, and the military utilize urine testing for drugs such as marijuana, cocaine, heroin, opiates generally, barbiturates, amphetamines, minor tranquilizers, PCP, LSD, and methaqualone. Tests are designed to measure either the parent drug or its metabolites (breakdown products). If the drug or its metabolite is found in the urine, it is safe to say that the person previously ingested the drug, either actively or passively. But *how* stoned, intoxicated, or impaired the person may or may not have been cannot be determined from the mere discovery of the drug in the urine.

How long can a drug be detected in the urine after the last dose is subject to at least seven variables: the drug itself, the size of the last dose, the length of time the drug was used, how the drug was taken, the number and chemical stability of its breakdown products in the body (metabolites), the solubility of the drug in the body fat, and the designed sensitivity of the procedure used to detect the drug. Major metabolites of marijuana can be detected in the urine of a heavy pot smoker a month after the last dose. Cocaine metabolites can be found after only about 4 days; amphetamines, heroin, and codeine, 1–2 days; and PCP, 7–14 days. All of these times are approximate and are subject to considerable individual variation.

Three methods are most often used to screen urine for drugs: thin-layer chromatography; the enzyme-multiplied immunoassay test (EMIT); and radioimmunoassay (RIA), an example of which is Abuscreen. Screening methods such as these are very accurate when done by trained personnel in analytical laboratories, but they are not intended to be the final answer. If they identify a positive urine sample, they must be confirmed by a more sensitive (and usually more expensive) procedure. Confirmation can be accomplished by gas chromatography, high-performance liquid chromatography, or a combination gas chromatography-mass spectroscopy. Cost for the initial screen can run $10–$60 per urine sample; confirmation can cost $100 or more per test.

The *chain of custody* of specimens in urine drug testing is of great practical and legal importance. One must be able to prove that the sample analyzed indeed came from the particular person. Chain of custody begins with the collection of the urine specimen and continues through transportation to the laboratory, handling during the analysis, and reporting of results. To be certain a particular person gave the sample, he or she must be observed urinating. The sample must be of body temperature, to prove that it was freshly voided. Samples and containers must be sealed and receipted. Authorized signatures are required at each custody in the chain. Any uncertainty in the chain of custody can be a basis for a court challenge of the test results. Under present law it is not a crime to have a controlled substance in your blood. Hence a positive test for a controlled substance in the urine is not a basis for a report to the police. Results of an employee's urine drug analysis must be kept private; employees must be protected against indiscriminate disclosure to third parties.

The laboratory conducting the analysis must decide on the cutoff concentration for reporting a positive result—that is, the amount of the drug the test sample must contain for the drug's presence to be important enough to mention. The choice of cutoff level will be governed by the sensitivity of the apparatus used, cost, and the medicolegal factors involved. If a testing laboratory errs and fails to report the presence of a drug in a urine sample, the result is termed a false negative. If the laboratory "finds" a drug that is not there, the result is a false positive. In the workplace setting it is the false positive that everyone is concerned about. A false positive can result, of course, from a laboratory error, but that is rare. It is more likely to be the result of other chemical substances in the person's blood—for example, a false positive for amphetamines could be given by a stimulant drug such as ephedrine or methylphenidate (Ritalin), or a diet drug containing phenylpropanolamine (examples: Acutrim, Appedrine, Control, Dexatrim, Permathene, Prolamine), or a decongestant product containing a sympathomimetic (examples: Alka-Seltzer Plus, Allerest, Bronkaid, Contac, Donnagel, NyQuil, Primateen, Sinutab, Sudafed, and Triaminic). Poppy seed cakes can give a false positive for morphine (this requires a very large ingestion of poppy seed); or a nonsteroidal anti-inflammatory drug such as ibuprofen (Advil) can give a false positive for marijuana. There has been criticism of the marijuana test allegedly because it discriminates against blacks, who have more melanin metabolites supposedly free-floating in their urine, where they can be mistaken for tetrahydrocannabinol (THC) metabolites. There is no substance to this criticism.

Additional false positives have been reported. In tests for barbiturates, Doriden, Nalton, and Dilantin have reported positive on screening tests. For opiates, Thorazine and dextromethorphan have reported positive. For phencyclidine (PCP),

Benadryl, Demerol, chlorpromazine, Mellaril, dextromethorphan, and Unisom have reported positive. For cocaine, coca leaf tea has reported positive.

In the case of false positives, confirmation tests can clear up the error. In fact, confirmation should be routine for any positive test obtained in an initial screen.

There is yet another kind of problem in drug testing, which is not a false positive but a false pitfall. Even your dear old sainted grandmother would have shown up positive for opiates if she had taken paregoric for diarrhea, Demerol or codeine for pain, or Lomotil or Vicks Formula 44. All of these substances are legally available over the counter or by prescription and contain an opiate or opioid (an opiumlike compound). You may have every right to be taking them, but your urine is going to show up positive, and you will either have to stop taking them a month in advance of the test or announce the fact of use to the test agency.

Is employee drug testing legal? The answer is that individuals acting as private citizens, and private employers, are not bound by Fourth Amendment constitutional restraints. Private employers may demand drug screening without violating the constitutional guarantee to privacy. While government employees are subject to the privacy and illegal search restrictions of the Constitution, urine testing by government employers has withstood recent challenges that it violates the Fourth Amendment.

For more information on individual drugs and their tests, see those sections.

See also DRUGS IN SPORTS, FALSE POSITIVE, MARIJUANA

Dulcolax

Bisacodyl, the active ingredient in this laxative, is also the active ingredient in Carter's Little Pills. See that section for a discussion of bisacodyl's undesirable features.

Because Dulcolax tablets are enteric-coated (designed to dissolve in the intestine and not in the stomach), they must be swallowed whole, not chewed. If the active ingredient is released into the stomach by mistake, it could cause vomiting.

Adverse effects: Abdominal cramping can be expected in some users after taking this product.

See also CARTER'S LITTLE PILLS

Duster

PCP comes in a powdered form called "angel dust." The powder can be mixed with marijuana (or parsley, mint, or oregano) and made into a marijuana cigarette (joint). Such joints are called dusters. Of course, when the joint is smoked, the PCP is volatilized and inhaled. PCP also comes in a liquid form. A cigarette dipped into the liquid PCP and allowed to dry is called a "sherm."

See also PCP

E

Emetrol

This OTC product is promoted for the treatment of nausea and vomiting. It contains fructose and glucose plus orthophosphoric acid in a pH-controlled mint-flavored solution.

The FDA has concluded that Emetrol lacks evidence of effectiveness as a treatment of nausea and vomiting. This is not too surprising because the "active" ingredients are very common substances. When table sugar (sucrose) is digested it gives the same two sugars, fructose and glucose.

If Emetrol appears to work in some people, the explanation might lie in the well-known placebo effect (see the section on placebos). Sometimes if we believe that a drug will work, it does—just because we have the expectation.

Ephedrine

Other name: none
Source: the plant *Ephedra trifurca,* chemical synthesis
Pharmacology: bronchodilator, nasal decongestant
Dose: orally, 15–50 mg; 1 EFED II capsule (yellow) contains

25 mg; Vatronol nose drops contain approximately 5 mg in each 20 drops

Ephedrine is the active ingredient in the plant *Ephedra tri-furca,* a shrub listed in the Chinese dispensatory as early as 1569. Ephedrine has long been used as a bronchodilator in the treatment of asthma, where it is given orally. However, its possible adverse effects are so serious that authorities today advise against its use in asthma. It also is a decongestant to the upper respiratory system, an action explained by its ability to constrict small blood vessels and reduce the volume of blood in tissues.

Ephedrine is a sympathomimetic drug, which means we can expect it to stimulate the heart and CNS. These actions can be unwanted side effects in its use as a bronchodilator. In fact, if you have heart disease, high blood pressure, an overactive thyroid gland, or diabetes, consult your physician before using ephedrine.

Misuse potential: medium

Adverse effects: Overdosage with ephedrine produces symptoms typical of sympathomimetics: restlessness, headache, heart palpitations, nausea, and possibly tremors.

Ephedrine is used in Wyanoids and Pazo hemorrhoidal suppositories supposedly for its vasoconstrictor effect. It is found in Primatene, Bronkaid, and Tedral asthma tablets, all of which the FDA has concluded lack evidence of safety and effectiveness in treating asthma.

Ephedrine has been used in look-alike drugs, especially speed look-alikes, where it is found in 12–25-mg doses (along with caffeine and phenylpropanolamine).

Drug interactions: The simultaneous use of monoamine oxidase inhibitor drugs and ephedrine can result in a dangerous hypertensive crisis. At least one death has been blamed on this combination. Ephedrine can diminish the effectiveness of dexamethasone and possibly other corticosteroids. It also can counteract the blood-pressure-lowering effects of guanethidine. Reserpine can reduce the effectiveness of ephedrine.

See also ADRENERGICS, ASTHMA PRODUCTS, LOOK-ALIKES, SYMPATHOMIMETICS

Epinephrine

Other names: Adrenalin, adrenaline, "epi"
Source: animal glands, synthesis
Pharmacology: sympathomimetic, heart stimulant, bronchodilator, vasoconstrictor (peripheral)
Dose: 0.3 mg; sprays of the Primatene and Bronkaid type typically deliver 0.2–0.3 mg of epinephrine per squeeze

In the human nervous system the point where one nerve ends and the next begins is called the synapse. A neurotransmitter is a chemical released from the end of the first nerve that helps the impulse cross the synapse and arrive at the next nerve. Of the great number of neurotransmitters in the human body, the four most important are epinephrine, norepinephrine, dopamine, and acetylcholine. The first three of these are termed catecholamines, and the parent compound is epinephrine. Catecholamines are released in the body when we are stressed, threatened, or made angry. Reactions to them constitute the "fight or flight" response. The major source of epinephrine is the adrenal gland.

Epinephrine is not only a neurotransmitter of great physiological importance, it also is a drug in its own right. As the quintessential sympathomimetic, it has actions on the cardiovascular system, bronchi, and other organs and tissues. It is used as a bronchodilator in asthma; to protect against hypersensitivity reactions to drugs and insect bites (some persons are so dangerously allergic to bee stings that they carry with them at all times a hypodermic syringe loaded with epinephrine); as a vasoconstrictor to prolong the action of infiltration anesthetics; and as a hemostatic agent to stop serious bleeding or hemorrhaging. Epinephrine is a powerful drug, having an average dose of only 0.3 mg.

Your doctor can prescribe larger doses of epinephrine for you, and he or she can discuss side effects or adverse effects with you. Epinephrine also is for sale OTC in the form of mists and inhalers for asthma. The OTC products are less potent, but since people tend to overuse them, their adverse effects can be every bit as real.

Products: Primatene Mist and Bronkaid Mist are sprays for inhalation that deliver epinephrine directly to the bronchi for treatment of acute asthma. Epipen Auto-Injector is designed for self-use by the layperson in case of insect stings, or food, drug, or other allergies. (CAUTION: For intramuscular use only; do not inject intravenously or into buttocks.)

Misuse potential: medium

Adverse effects: Epinephrine is a powerful stimulant to the brain and cardiovascular system. Even ordinary doses of it can cause restlessness, insomnia, and rapid heartbeat. If these symptoms occur while using an epinephrine-type product, reduce the dose or discontinue the drug. If you have diabetes, high blood pressure, or thyroid disease, do not use epinephrine products without first consulting your physician. If you are pregnant or nursing a baby, see your doctor before using this drug. Do not use in children under 6 years of age. If you use an epinephrine mist for asthma and do not obtain relief in the first 20–30 minutes, stop using the drug and get immediate medical attention. Hyperthyroid patients and those with heart disease or hypertension are not good candidates for epinephrine therapy. If there is a choice, avoid the use of this drug in aged persons. Epinephrine's adverse effects can include heart palpitation, dizziness, weakness, headache, throbbing, anxiety, fear, and breathing difficulty.

Drug interactions: Epinephrine's effects can be dangerously potentiated by tricyclic antidepressants such as Elavil and by certain antihistamines. Diabetes mellitus patients should know that epinephrine can raise blood sugar levels and thus necessitate a change in dose of insulin.

See also ASTHMA PRODUCTS, SYMPATHOMIMETICS

Ergot

Other names for active ingredient: ergot alkaloids, ergotamine

Source: the fungus *Claviceps purpurea*

Pharmacology: vasoconstrictor, uterine stimulant, for treating senile mental decline, migraine

Dose: typically, 1 tablet (containing 0.5–1.0 mg)

Ergot is a fungal parasite that grows on and contaminates rye and other cereal grains. It can grow anywhere in the world, but the most recent outbreak of ergotism occurred in Ethiopia in 1978.

Ergot contains the ergot alkaloids, of which ergotamine is best known, as it is used medicinally in Cafergot, a treatment for migraine headaches. The ergot alkaloids possess a powerful vasoconstrictor action, believed to be the basis for their action in migraine (the theory is that expanded blood vessels in the brain cause the headaches). However, this same vasoconstrictor action makes ergotamine a dangerous drug to use without supervision, and more than one patient has suffered gangrene of the extremities from unsupervised, lengthy use of ergot.

The ergot alkaloids can also powerfully contract the uterus (womb). Although in years past this property was used in illegal abortions, today ergot alkaloids are used after delivery to control bleeding.

It is of considerable interest that all of the ergot alkaloids are derivatives of lysergic acid; hydrolysis of the alkaloid liberates the lysergic acid. In 1938 Hofmann in Switzerland first prepared the N,N-diethylamide derivative of lysergic acid, now known as the hallucinogen LSD.

Products: Cafergot tablets contain 1 mg of ergotamine tartrate and 100 mg of caffeine; suppositories are available that contain 2 mg of ergotamine and 100 mg of caffeine. Cafergot is intended to abort or prevent vascular (migraine) headaches. Bellergal, Ergostat, and Wigraine are similar preparations. Medihaler Ergotamine is an aerosol for inhaling a fine-particle suspension of ergotamine tartrate as a rapid treatment of migraine. Hydergine is a preparation of ergot alkaloids promoted for use in people over 60 who show signs of declining mental capacity.

Abuse potential: low

Adverse effects: The ergot alkaloids, whether found alone or in combination with drugs such as caffeine, are potent drugs that must be used only under a doctor's direct supervision. Never increase the dose or take for longer than prescribed. Because of their powerful vasoconstrictor action, the ergot alkaloids can diminish or even stop circulation in the fingers, toes, arms, or legs. If you feel numbness or tingling, or observe signs of cyanosis (blue color), stop taking the drug immediately and get immediate medical attention. Ergot alkaloids can cause vomiting, diarrhea, weakness in the legs, localized redness, and itching. WARNING: Pregnant women should consult their doctor before using any ergot preparation.

Drug interactions: A dangerous vasoconstriction leading to gangrene can develop if ergot alkaloids are administered together with dopamine; there is some evidence that Inderal can produce the same effect. They should be used with extreme caution in patients with severe vascular disease. CAUTION: Ergot alkaloids are very potent drugs and must be used only under constant medical supervision. They should never be given to pregnant women or those about to become pregnant.

See also MIGRAINE

Estrogen

Other names: estradiol, estriol, estrone, Premarin
Source: pregnant human and animal urines, synthesis
Pharmacology: female sex hormones
Dose: 0.01–2.5 mg; Premarin tablets are supplied in strengths of 0.3, 0.625, 0.9, 1.25, and 2.5 mg.

The estrogenic hormones make the difference between a prepubertal girl and a postadolescent woman. All the secondary sex characteristics that develop in females are based, in some measure, upon the secretion and action of the natural estrogens estradiol, estriol, and estrone. Estrogens help develop and maintain the female reproductive system—that is, the vagina, uterus, and Fallopian tubes. They are important in breast enlargement, shape of the female body, long bone growth, body hair, and pigmentation of the nipples and genitals. They play an important role in the female psyche. Estrogen levels are a key factor in the menstrual cycle. Menopause marks the time of gradual termination of estrogen secretion in females, and therefore estrogen replacement therapy becomes an important consideration.

CAUTION: Estrogens are very potent hormones. They should NOT be used during pregnancy. They should be used on a physician's prescription and should never be given to a friend who has not seen a physician for advice.

If natural estrogen levels are too low or are absent, outside (exogenous) estrogen can be prescribed. This can be obtained from pregnant human or mares' urine or by synthesis. Horses produce large amounts of estrogens that are similar enough in chemical structure to work very well in the human. Exogenous estrogen is widely used today to treat women suffering through the menopause, for senile vaginitis, failure of ovarian development, and for acne (in both males and females). Of course, estrogen is widely used in the combination oral contraceptive pill.

Estrogen-containing creams are available on prescription for direct vaginal application in menopausal women. Transdermal estradiol (that is, skin patch application), now approved by the FDA, offers advantages over the oral route, since oral estrogen is partly destroyed in the GI tract. Also, oral estrogen is more likely to induce enzyme systems in the liver and to increase the risk of blood clots. Estraderm from Ciba-Geigy is estrogen in skin patch form.

Estrogen in skin creams and cosmetics is widely promoted as an agent to delay or correct the effects of aging, but there is no scientific evidence that you are getting your money's worth. No cosmetic on the market can reverse the effects of aging. Recently the FDA warned 11 firms that market anti-aging products that they must cease and desist misleading advertising or risk seizure of their products.

There is a danger in applying estrogen to the skin, and that is the very good possibility that estrogen will be absorbed into the bloodstream and be circulated to all body parts, where it can have significant side effects. For example, breast enlargement was seen in a 10-month-old girl and in a 5-year-old boy on whom estrogen hair creams had been used. An 82-year-old woman and a 54-year-old man had side effects after a hair lotion containing estrogen had been used, and an 8-month-old girl began to develop breasts after her diaper rash was treated with an estrogen product. Remember: Estrogens are hormones, and they are powerfully active in milligram doses. If you are using a cosmetic containing a "hormone," check it out with a pharmacist.

Misuse potential: medium

Adverse effects: Never take any estrogen product (including an oral contraceptive) if you are pregnant, or even if you suspect you are pregnant. There is sufficient evidence to conclude that estrogen causes birth defects; even a few doses could be disastrous for your fetus.

Today there is controversy about the safety of exogenous estrogen. Estrogens and endometrial cancer have been linked in various research studies carried out over the past eight years (the endometrium is the inner lining of the uterus). In each of these studies women with endometrial cancer were compared with equal numbers of controls matched for age, area of residence, and intact uterus. Each study showed that the women with endometrial cancer had a greater history of estrogen use than the controls. In one study nearly half of the cancer patients were estrogen users, whereas only about one sixth of the controls were. This finding is not proof, but it is accepted as strong epidemiologic evidence upon which the *risk* of estrogen use is based.

Ayerst Laboratories, the manufacturer of Premarin, publishes prescribing information that is directed to the physician and prospective user. Ayerst says that independent case studies show a 4.5 to 13.9 times greater risk of endometrial cancer in postmenopausal women exposed to exogenous estrogen for more than 1 year. This risk is further substantiated by the discovery that incidence rates of endometrial cancer have risen sharply since 1969 in eight areas of the United States that have population-based cancer-reporting systems. The increased incidence could be related to the growing use of estrogen in past decades.

The FDA upon review of studies of estrogen use has concluded that menopausal and postmenopausal women who take estrogens have an increased risk of uterine cancer. This risk is proportional to the duration of estrogen use and is particularly high with use of 5 years or longer. The FDA has published the following advice concerning the risks and benefits of estrogen therapy:

> The usefulness of estrogens in treating certain symptoms of the menopause . . . is well established. In most women undergoing menopause, however, if psychosomatic and anxiety symptoms predominate, these can often be managed with reassurance and, if necessary, with anti-anxiety medications. . . . Estrogens are obviously used to a far greater extent and for a longer time, however, than can be accounted for by the incidence or duration of acute menopausal symptoms . . . estrogen use appears to exceed by far that required for short-term management of the menopausal syndrome.

NOTE: In some people, the benefits of estrogen use can greatly outweigh any risks—for example, in the treatment of osteoporosis. Your physician can help you weigh the decision of whether or not to take estrogens.

Drug interactions: Phenobarbital speeds up the body's destruction of estrogens; the two should not be mixed. Ampicillin may negate the effects of oral contraceptives containing estrogen. Diabetics taking antidiabetic drugs should monitor carefully their blood sugar levels if they are also taking estrogen products.

See also ACNE TREATMENTS, DIETHYLSTILBESTROL

Excedrin

Other names of active ingredients: aspirin, acetaminophen, caffeine

Source: compounding

Pharmacology: pain and fever reliever

Dose: each tablet or capsule contains 250 mg of both aspirin and acetaminophen, plus 65 mg of caffeine

This product contains *both* aspirin and acetaminophen, an irrational combination because taken together these 2 painkillers are no more effective than taken singly, but by ingesting both you risk the side effects of both. What is more, Excedrin contains caffeine—a stimulant that can cause sleeplessness, heart arrhythmias, and tremors. The FDA has ruled that for treating headaches, caffeine does not show evidence of being safe and effective. Caffeine will not relieve the pain of arthritis, sore muscles, or sore throat.

Excedrin P.M. contains acetaminophen and the antihistamine diphenhydramine. The FDA has ruled that there is no evidence that diphenhydramine is a safe and effective drug for the treatment of pain. Antihistamines are useful for the treatment of allergies, and they do help some people get to sleep. It would appear wise that if insomnia is your problem, you could take just a hypnotic (sleep-inducing) drug and not expose yourself to another drug you don't need. Generic acetaminophen must conform to the same USP standards as the acetaminophen in Excedrin, and the cost of the generic can be as much as two thirds less.

Excedrin is an expensive product. All of its active ingredients can be purchased individually and generically.

Misuse potential: medium

Adverse effects: Aspirin can irritate the lining of the stomach. It can interfere with the clotting of the blood and should never be used by ulcer patients, pregnant women, or those contemplating surgery. Do not use aspirin products after a tonsillectomy. A very small percentage of the population may be highly sensitive (or allergic) to aspirin, suffering pain, shock, or even death from one dose. There is no sure way to predict who will experience such a reaction to aspirin, but it is known that asthmatics are far more susceptible to an attack than nonasthmatics. Aspirin can cause skin rash, kidney damage, changes in blood cells, and upset stomach in sensitive users.

Acetaminophen probably will not cause you any significant adverse effects if you do not exceed the recommended dosage. However, excessive doses can lead to liver damage. The kidney is also sensitive to overdosage. CAUTION: Persons with a history of liver disease should avoid excessive use of acetaminophen and should restrict its use to brief periods.

Caffeine produces few adverse effects in most people, but sensitive users may find it difficult to get to sleep after ingesting caffeine. Heavy doses can cause the heart to beat irregularly or cause shakiness and irritability. There is some evidence that caffeine can cause birth defects, but the FDA has not agreed with such a conclusion. There is also some evidence that links caffeine to the occurrence of fibrocystic breast disease (noncancerous lumps in the breast).

Drug interactions: Aspirin interactions are common. Combined with alcohol or with an anticoagulant, it can dangerously increase bleeding tendency. Aspirin taken concurrently with Orinase, Diabinese, or other oral antidiabetic drugs can cause too great a lowering of blood sugar. Aspirin will antagonize the systemic reactions of the anti-arthritic drugs Anturane and Benemid. If you are taking *any* prescription medication, talk to your doctor before heavily dosing yourself with aspirin.

Acetaminophen can intensify the effects of concurrently administered oral anticoagulants. Combining alcohol with acetaminophen can increase the poisonous effects of both on the liver. Either avoid these drug combinations or consult your doctor beforehand.

See also ACETAMINOPHEN, ASPIRIN, CAFFEINE, GENERIC DRUGS

F

False Negative

If, in the testing for the presence of a drug or chemical in body fluids or anywhere else, the test fails to show the presence of the drug or chemical, the result is said to be a false negative.

False negative results can be due to errors in the planning and execution of the test procedure or to the presence of interfering substances. False negatives are especially undesirable if they permit drug use to go undetected or if they fail to show a pregnancy in the continued use of an oral contraceptive (because of the danger of birth defects).

Tests for sugar in the urine, phenylketonuria (PKU), and ketoacidosis can be carried out by the layperson at home by use of the handy "dip and read" products commercially available. Users of these products must carefully follow the directions to avoid false readings.

See also DRUGS, TESTING FOR; FALSE POSITIVE

False Positive

If, in the laboratory testing for the presence of a drug or chemical in body fluids or anywhere else, the procedure gives a result that indicates the drug or chemical is present when in actuality it is not, the result is termed a false positive. False positives can result, of course, from a careless or flawed testing procedure, but that is rare. They are more likely to result from the unexpected presence of an interfering drug or chemical—one that behaves the same in the test. See the section on drug testing for examples. False results can result from samples that have been switched deliberately or accidentally.

Modern laboratories build systems of checks and balances into their procedures to thwart analytical errors before results are reported. For many, a false positive is more unfortunate than a false negative because it can result in unjustified legal or personal action against an individual. Passive inhalation of marijuana smoke can produce blood levels of tetrahydrocannabinol high enough to be detected by very sensitive procedures. In a way this could be considered a false positive.

Examples of drug interactions that can result in false positives or false negatives are: Massive doses of penicillin can cause a false positive test for sugar in the urine; aspirin or other salicylates can cause a false negative test for sugar in the urine; inhaled nasal decongestants can be absorbed, appear in the urine, and give a false positive test for catecholamines; ephedrine, Ritalin, and antiobesity drugs can give false positives for amphetamines; Dilantin can give a false positive for barbiturates; dextromethorphan can yield a false positive for opiates.

False positives and false negatives are greatly reduced when confirmatory tests are carried out, and that is the general procedure in modern laboratories.

See also DRUGS, TESTING FOR

Fentanyl

Other names: Sublimaze injection, Innovar injection
Source: synthesis
Pharmacology: nacrotic analgesic
Dose: 0.1 mg. Available only in ampules for injection. Each milliliter supplies 0.05 mg.

In the same category as morphine and meperidine, fentanyl is a narcotic analgesic, but it is some 100 times more powerful than morphine and about 750 times more potent than meperidine in pain relief. Marketed as Sublimaze, it is now used in an estimated 70% of all surgeries in the United States. It has gained a reputation as a safe and effective drug, although it can depress respiration dangerously and slow the heart. It appears to cause less nausea and vomiting than morphine and codeine. Its duration of action is quite brief: 30–60 minutes after a single injection of 0.1 mg.

Abuse potential: high. Sublimaze is very widely used in hospitals across the country; some physicians and other health professionals have become dependent on it. Fentanyl, itself a controlled substance, has become the chemical model for the creation of analogs, or "designer drugs," by which unscrupulous chemists hope to evade the Controlled Substances Act and make a lot of money. (Until a compound is classified or "scheduled," no laws apply to it.) The first analog of fentanyl, alpha-methylfentanyl, was uncovered in 1979 in Orange City, California, and was found to be 200 times more potent than morphine. Since then, almost a dozen other analogs have appeared on the streets, including para-fluorofentanyl and the infamous 3-methylfentanyl.

Since fentanyl analogs are so powerful and their dose so small, only tiny amounts of them will occur in body fluids, and this makes testing for them very difficult. Further, fentanyl analogs do not give positive urine tests for opiates. The street drug "China White" has been identified in one report as 3-methylfentanyl.

Adverse effects: As a typical narcotic analgesic, fentanyl depresses respiration; big enough doses can stop breathing altogether. Fentanyl can cause a large drop in blood pressure, nausea, sweating, dizziness, and blurred vision.

Drug interactions: Combined with barbiturates, tranquilizers, or other brain depressants, fentanyl can cause too great a sedation of the brain. The use of Sublimaze with monoamine oxidase inhibitors is not recommended.

See also NARCOTIC ANALGESICS

G

Gasoline. *See* SOLVENTS AND INHALANTS

Gelusil. *See* ANTACIDS

Ginseng

Other name: Panax
Source: plant root
Pharmacology: purported tonic and stimulant
Dose: not used in American medicine

Ginseng has been used by the Chinese for thousands of years. They regard it as a tonic and stimulant that can restore the forces of *yin* and *yang* to their proper balance. Korean ginseng is sold in the United States as pills, capsules, or the powdered root.

Ginseng is not official in the *U.S. Pharmacopoeia* and is not considered to be a useful drug by American doctors. However, it carries a reputation in other circles as a cure for convulsions, dizziness, nervous disorders, colds, fever, headache, shortness of breath, and as an agent to stop bleeding from wounds. Some believe it to be an antidote to stress and a mildly active sexual stimulant (in doses of 1 g a day). The mere fact that it is supposed to accomplish so many cures, of course, makes one suspicious that it can accomplish any real cures.

Ginseng does not appear to be dangerous to use, and if you have no success using it as a tonic of some sort the most you could be wasting is your money.

Glue Sniffing. *See* SOLVENTS AND INHALANTS

Glutethimide

Other name: Doriden
Source: synthesis
Pharmacology: CNS depressant, sleep-inducer
Dose: 0.25–0.50 g at bedtime for insomnia. (Both 0.25 and 0.50 g tablets are available.) For the aged or debilitated patient the initial dose should not exceed 0.125–0.25 g at bedtime.

Introduced in 1954 as a sedative-hypnotic drug and marketed extensively as Doriden, this CNS depressant is another example of a nonbarbiturate that has been abused. The manufacturers make it clear that for sleep induction Doriden should be used for 3 to 7 days only. Use for longer periods can clearly lead to tolerance, dependence, and a withdrawal syndrome that can involve epileptic seizures. A psychological dependence can also develop in which there is no physical reliance but a psychic need to continue the drug. Because large doses of glutethimide can be fatal, the drug has a history of use in suicide attempts. Actually, many physicians will no longer prescribe glutethimide because better, less toxic drugs have become available.

Glutethimide is one of a group of loosely related nonbarbiturate sedative-hypnotics, the members of which have gained considerable notoriety. The group includes Noludar (methyprylon), Quaalude (methaqualone, now banned), Placidyl (ethchlorvynol), and Valmid (ethinamate). These are discussed in their own sections in this book.

In the 1960s glutethimide became a street drug of abuse, and numerous cases of addiction were identified. As usual, this led to tighter controls and more restrictive distribution. In retrospect, glutethimide's abuse potential could have been predicted based upon its chemical and pharmacological similarity to the barbiturates.

Abuse potential: high

Adverse effects: Users of glutethimide occasionally report nausea, a kind of next-morning hangover, blurring of vision, and infrequently a paradoxical excitation. Long-term users show chronic toxicity signs, including tremors, loss of memory, slurring of speech, and general depression. WARNING: Driving a car or operating machinery while under the influence of Doriden can be hazardous. The most serious adverse effect of

Doriden is its ability to induce tolerance and physical dependence in persons who use it for weeks or months, especially if
they are taking large doses. Reliance on pills to get to sleep is
unwise in the first place, and much more so if the drug is in the
glutethimide category.

Drug interactions: Combining Doriden with other CNS
depressants, especially alcohol, can result in overdepression of
the CNS. When a person receiving oral anticoagulants is started
on glutethimide or stopped, the anticoagulant dosage may have
to be adjusted.

See also BARBITURATES

Growth Hormone

Other names: HGH, Humatrope, Protropin
Sources: gene splicing, human cadavers
Pharmacology: growth and metabolism regulator
Dose: variable, typically 2–5 mg given 3 times weekly for 1
year

Until recently, if a child was not growing at a normal rate or
was clearly diagnosed as a pituitary dwarf, the only agent that
could be given to ensure at least a reasonable growth was
human growth hormone (HGH), obtained from the pituitary
glands of cadavers. No other animal growth hormone was suf-
ficiently similar to substitute in the human. Since the supply of
HGH was very limited, not every child who needed it received
it. Also, because of the possibility of AIDS virus transmission (or
other agents such as Cruetzfeldt-Jakob virus) in and with the
preparation, human HGH was less than the ideal treatment.

Now all that has changed. Gene-spliced HGH now is available
from two firms: Genentech markets Protropin, and Eli Lilly has
received FDA approval to market Humatrope. Although it contains the same sequence of 191 amino acids as found in natural
HGH, Protropin differs in having an extra methionine on the
nitrogen-terminus of the molecule. Lilly's Humatrope is exactly
the same as natural human HGH.

These gene-spliced hormones (also termed recombinant
DNA hormones) are to be used only for long-term treatment of
children whose pituitary glands are not producing enough natural HGH to ensure a reasonable stature. Along with height, the

hormone affects cell growth and metabolism of carbohydrates, proteins, fats, and minerals.

The cost of treating each case of hypopituitary dwarfism is $8000 worth of Protropin a year. While Protropin has been shown to double or triple the growth rate of hormone-deficient babies, there is no evidence that it will induce normal children to grow taller.

Abuse potential: medium. Weight lifters, football linemen, and other athletes who want to gain a competitive edge have been taking HGH. Its use extends from professional teams to high schoolers and apparently to most all nations of the world. It is very difficult to detect exogenous HGH, since it is found normally in the bodies of healthy people. To thwart the black market in HGH that seems to be developing, the makers of gene-spliced HGH will distribute it only to selected medical centers in the United States. However, there is ample evidence that HGH is entering this country from foreign sources.

Adverse effects: Physicians have learned the adverse effects of too much HGH from observing pituitary giants—people born with a grossly overactive pituitary gland. Acromegaly results, a condition in which the jaw and forehead grow out of proportion. Teeth become widely separated, fingers and toes swell, and there is redness, pain, vomiting, and headache. Athletes who have used HGH heavily for months or years have experienced heart attacks. It is generally conceded that the abuser of HGH will have a shorter life-span.

See also DRUGS IN SPORTS

Guarana

Other name of active ingredient: caffeine
Source: herb
Pharmacology: brain and heart stimulant; diuretic
Dose: variable

Guarana has been a hot sales item recently, especially on the West Coast. It is prepared from a plant native to Brazil, and it has an unusually high caffeine content—far more than coffee. In Brazil it is the national drink and often is made into sweet, carbonated beverages.

Unscrupulous dealers pass off guarana as cocaine, or at least some powerful, illicit CNS stimulant, and the neophyte falls for the deception because of the very high caffeine content. Guarana is also sold truthfully labeled as a tonic stimulant to bring you up to your "best." It is an expensive way to obtain the same caffeine found in a cup or two of coffee.

Abuse potential: medium

Adverse effects: Most normal, healthy people will experience few if any adverse effects from the caffeine in guarana, but sensitive users may find it difficult to get to sleep after taking this drug. Heavy doses of caffeine can cause the heart to beat irregularly or cause shakiness and irritability. Certain consumer groups claim that caffeine causes birth defects, but the FDA has not agreed with that conclusion. There also is some evidence that links caffeine to the occurrence of fibrocystic breast disease (noncancerous lumps in the breast).

Drug interactions: If caffeine is combined with a monoamine oxidase inhibitor such as Parnate or Nardil, dangerously high blood pressure may result. Caffeine may increase the effects of thyroid drugs and amphetamines but cancel the calming effects of barbiturates and other sedatives.

See also CAFFEINE

H

Hallucinogenic Amphetamine Derivatives

Other names: MDA, MDM (MDMA, XTC, ADAM), MMDA, STP (DOM), TMA

Source: synthesis

Pharmacology: hallucinogens, psychomotor stimulants, euphoriants

Dose: see following table

Since the late 1960s, people seeking the chemical pursuit of ecstasy have taken any of a half-dozen drugs that are closely related chemically to the amphetamines. Because these compounds have a special stimulatory effect on the brain, they are termed hallucinogenic amphetamines. Their symbols, names, and doses are given in the following table:

Symbol	Chemical Name	Effective Hallucinogenic Dose
MDA	3,4-methylenedioxyamphetamine	50–150 mg
MDM (or, MDMA, XTC, ADAM, E)	N-methyl-3,4-methylenedioxyamphetamine (or methylenedioxymethamphetamine)	50–150 mg
MMDA	3-methoxy-4,5-methylenedioxyamphetamine	—
STP (DOM)	4-methyl-2,5-dimethoxyamphetamine	10 mg maximum
TMA	3,4,5-trimethoxyamphetamine (or, alpha-methylmescaline)	—

MDA first appeared in San Francisco during the 1967 "Summer of Love" and gained a reputation for eliciting a sensual, easily managed euphoria. But then the "Mellow Drug of America" lost its appeal and has largely been replaced by its close chemical relative MDMA (also known as Ecstasy, XTC, MDM). Both drugs are modified amphetamines and can cause muscle tension, sweating, insomnia, tremors, a fast heart rate, and paranoia. But it is for their psychic effects that they have become popular street drugs. They induce a feeling of peace, openness, insight, delight, self-awareness, and hallucination. Some users take MDMA all day for its CNS stimulant euphoric effects, or as an aphrodisiac. Hundreds of thousands of doses of MDMA are being sold on the street, typically as a white powder costing about $50 a gram. It can be inhaled, injected, or swallowed.

Both MDA and MDM have now been placed on Schedule I of the Controlled Substances Act, and possession of either is potentially a felony. However, before this scheduling was made, MDM gained the respectability of therapeutic use by psychiatrists treating depressed people. Dozens of therapists reported good results in many cases.

The DEA considers both MDA and MDM to be dangerous drugs that can cause a long-lasting reduction in the brain's supply of serotonin. An MDA dose of 7.5 mg per kilogram of body weight in humans is close to the lethal dose. One study showed that some 90% of MDA/MDM street samples are authentic.

STP has gained an aura of mystery, since no one really knows what the initials stand for. Achieving notoriety in the summer of 1967, STP got the reputation of being a powerful CNS stimulant capable of causing auditory and visual hallucinations, telepathic powers, and a euphoria lasting for up to 14 hours. It is less popular today, possibly because of its high incidence of bad trips. STP is a synthetic substance, active in doses of a few milligrams. On a weight basis, therefore, it is about one tenth as active as LSD.

Knowing that STP is an amphetamine, we could have predicted many of its pharmacological effects: an increase in heart rate and blood pressure, dilation of the pupil of the eye, bronchodilation, decreased appetite, and CNS stimulation.

Abuse potential: high for all examples

Adverse effects: Chemical dependency is the most serious threat in the use of these drugs. Users come to depend upon the feelings of peace, insight, openness, and self-awareness they experience from these amphetamine derivatives. They term MDMA a consciousness-effective drug. Because these drugs are sympathomimetics related to amphetamine, they should not be used by anyone with high blood pressure, heart or cardiovascular disease, diabetes, or hypoglycemia. If you have a history of seizures, stay away from these drugs. Breast-feeding mothers and women who are pregnant or think they are pregnant should not ingest any of these drugs. Users should not attempt to drive a car or use machinery even though they think they are perfectly capable of doing so. Severe, day-long panic and anxiety attacks have been attributed to DOM.

Drug interactions: It is critical that these drugs not be combined with monoamine oxidase inhibitors such as Parnate or Nardil, because dangerously high blood pressure could result. Combining any of these drugs with amphetamines or any other brain stimulant could result in dangerous overstimulation.

See also AMPHETAMINES

Hallucinogens

Hallucinogens are chemicals that in small doses produce changes in perception, thought, and mood. They make people see and hear things that are not there.

Probably the most famous hallucinogen is LSD, but before it, the native populations of the world had psilocybin and psilocin (from Mexican mushrooms), ololiuqui, cohoba, harmala alkaloids, scopolamine, and mescaline (peyote).

There is a range of hallucinogenic effects produced by drugs. LSD is a powerful agent, producing visual and auditory hallucinations so intense as to mimic a psychotic state. Marijuana, most users say, produces at best mild effects. There is also a wide range of drugs that are hallucinogens, representing many different kinds of chemical structures as complex as the indolethylamines and as simple as dimethylformamide. With this diversity it is next to impossible to explain exactly how hallucinogens cause their mind-altering effects.

The response to a hallucinogen can be influenced by *set* and *setting*—that is, the set of one's mind (anticipation or dread), and the setting (environment, presence of companions). Bad trips or "bummers" can occur, with the entire psychedelic experience a dreadful ordeal. Others have "tripped" hundreds of times and are ready for more.

All of the hallucinogens are CNS stimulants; they increase brain activity and wakefulness, and they induce the typical "fight or flight" response. Often tolerance to a hallucinogen develops. LSD users must refrain from the drug for 3 to 5 days before it can act on them again.

All of the famous hallucinogens—LSD, mescaline, psilocybin, harmala—are Schedule I drugs, which means that the Drug Enforcement Administration considers them dangerous, high-abuse potential drugs and has made their possession or sale illegal and punishable with fines and/or jail sentences.

Abuse potential: high

Adverse effects: Many tens of thousands of hallucinogenic "trips" have been taken over the past 30 years, most under the influence of LSD. Early on it was noted that in certain sensitive people psychotic breaks could be precipitated by the hallucinogen. In others the experience was termed a "bummer"—that is, there were unpleasant, disturbing, even psychotic episodes that made the person believe he or she was losing their mind. LSD also produces physical effects: dilated pupil, flushed face, chilliness, a rise in body temperature, increase in heart rate, goose bumps, salivation, and perspiration. In the long term, LSD is well known for producing flashbacks in a small percentage of users. In this phenomenon the user spontaneously reexperiences LSD-like symptoms weeks or months after the last dose was taken. There is no way to stop the flashback, which may involve considerable dread and panic. People do not become physically dependent on LSD but can become psychologically dependent.

Drug interactions: Concurrent use of epinephrine, dopamine, or brain stimulants such as the amphetamines or hallucinogenic amphetamine derivatives can induce a dangerous psychotic state.

See also LSD, HALLUCINOGENIC AMPHETAMINE DERIVATIVES, MESCALINE, MUSHROOMS, PSYCHEDELICS

Hashish

Other name: hemp resin
Source: the plant *Cannabis sativa*
Pharmacology: psychoactive
Dose: variable

The marijuana plant, *Cannabis sativa,* also known as hemp, is the source of the tetrahydrocannabinols. The intoxicating effects of the tetrahydrocannabinols are discussed in the section on marijuana.

The highest concentration of tetrahydrocannabinols in marijuana is found in the plant's resin, and the highest concentration of resin in found in flowering tops of the female plants. The resin itself can be gathered and pressed into lumps or cakes. We term this hashish. When the resin is extracted and the solvent removed to form a thick, black liquid, the product is termed hash oil. Hashish or hash oil usually are smoked but also can be eaten.

Abuse potential: high
Adverse effects: The concentration of tetrahydrocannabinols in these products is far greater than in marijuana. Hashish con-

tains 10–20% and hash oil 30–40%. It is far easier to get "stoned" on these concentrated forms. Driving a car under the influence of tetrahydrocannabinols is dangerous at any time, but especially after using hashish or hash oil.

Drug interactions: Marijuana is a mild hallucinogen; combining other mind-altering drugs with it can increase the effects of both. It also is a brain depressant; combining alcohol with it can produce oversedation.

See also MARIJUANA

HCG

Other name: human chorionic gonadotropin

Source: human urine, gene splicing

Pharmacology: hormone of pregnancy; basis for home pregnancy test

Dose: not applicable

Weight reduction clinics are unlikely places to encounter HCG, but that is exactly where many women today use this substance as a drug. HCG is promoted in such clinics as a substance that, when injected, hastens the loss of body fat (used, of course, as part of an ongoing overall treatment regimen). Women who have taken HCG for weight reduction confirm the clinics' claims. Representatives of the FDA, however, state that there is absolutely no rational application of this hormone of pregnancy in weight reduction. Medical authorities state that HCG has no known effect on fat mobilization, on appetite or sense of hunger, or on body fat distribution; they believe it to be ineffective in causing a more attractive or normal distribution of fat. In 1977 the FDA reported on a controlled clinical study of 200 patients at Lackland Air Force Base in Texas. The study compared the effectiveness of HCG and a placebo in a weight reduction program. The patients given HCG lost an average of 15.0 pounds; those given the placebo lost an average of 15.4 pounds.

HCG is indeed a vital hormone of pregnancy. This glycoprotein, secreted by the placenta soon after conception, stimulates the corpus luteum to enlarge and secrete progesterone for maintenance of the pregnancy. Gynecologists administer HCG to infertile women, in conjunction with FSH and LH, to induce ovulation. Chorionic gonadotropins for injection *USP* is made from the urine of pregnant women and is marketed as A.P.L., Glukor Injection, Profasi HP, and others.

HCG detection in the urine is a recently developed, inexpensive (less than $10) test for pregnancy and can be purchased without a prescription. Some examples of trade products are E.P.T., Answer, Predictor, and Daisy 2. The manufacturers state that these products can be used at home to detect pregnancy as early as 9 days after the date the last menstrual period was expected to begin. Research has shown that by the ninth day there usually is sufficient HCG in the urine of a pregnant woman to be detected by the sensitive color test developed for this purpose. The manufacturers claim that their pregnancy tests are accurate 97% of the time when a positive result indicates that the woman is pregnant. But critics point out that when the test result shows that the woman is not pregnant, the test may be wrong as much as 20% of the time. In other words, there are many more false negatives than false positives.

HCG has been made by recombinant DNA technology at Integrated Genetics, Inc., Framingham, Massachusetts.

Misuse potential: medium (in weight-reduction clinics)

Adverse effects: HCG can stimulate the development of secondary sex characteristics in the male, and thus precocious puberty sometimes is seen in boys given this drug. Edema (the abnormal accumulation of body water) can occur, as can headache, tiredness, restlessness, and irritability.

Head Shop

A head shop is a store that specializes in the sale of drug paraphernalia. In many states and localities laws now forbid head shops, but elsewhere they continue to offer bongs (water pipes); literature for growing, preparing, or doing "your own"; seeds; conversion kits; magazines; and containers for storing drugs. They do not actually sell controlled substances but might have some "practice pot" for sale. The name "head" refers to a person who uses psychoactive drugs, especially marijuana (pot head) or LSD (acid head).

Drug paraphernalia are also widely offered for sale by mail order companies; they advertise in certain magazines. One ad offered an expensive conversion kit that would supposedly isomerize delta-8-tetrahydrocannabinol (found in marijuana) to the more psychoactive delta-9 isomer.

Heet. *See* COUNTERIRRITANTS

Hemorrhoidal Products

There is much misleading advertising in the area of hemorrhoidal products. Preparation H contains "active" ingredients that the experts say don't work (see the section on Preparation H). Other products may temporarily relieve symptoms but offer no cure. In fact, they may be harmful for you because they help you put off needed medical attention. In some cases an allergy to the dubious medication may develop. In the area of hemorrhoidal treatment, you are much better off seeking and heeding medical advice than paying attention to the ads.

Hemorrhoids (also termed piles) are bulging or dilated blood vessels and supporting tissues in the anal region. Complications include blood clots from ruptures of hemorrhoidal veins, "skin tabs" (fibrous connective tissue covered by anal skin), and prolapsed hemorrhoids (protusion of tissue through the anal opening).

People get hemorrhoids because of a genetic predisposition, their occupational status, or generally because of the human upright position.

Hemorrhoids can cause pain, itching, swelling, burning, and irritation, and it is to relieve these symptoms that people take the numerous OTC products that are available. However, hemorrhoids usually cannot be cured by self-treatment, and sometimes there are other causes for the anorectal symptoms. For example, inflammation, pain, and bleeding can be caused by a bacterial infection, an anal fistula, cryptitis, cancer, secondary lesions of syphilis, pinworms, or polyps (benign tumors of the bowel). The advice of a physician is required for these conditions. If hemorrhoidal symptoms do not improve after 7 days, a physician should be consulted.

The following table summarizes the active ingredients found in some OTC hemorrhoidal products and provides information about each type:

Type of Ingredient	Examples	Comments
protectant	zinc oxide, cocoa butter, mineral oil, cod liver oil, calamine, petrolatum	Form a barrier or protective cover. Reduce irritation. Do not cure.
local anesthetic	benzocaine, pramoxine (used topically)	Can relieve pain but do not heal. Allergic reactions to benzocaine can develop.
vasoconstrictor	ephedrine, epinephrine, phenylephrine	Supposedly constrict swollen blood vessels, but there is no good evidence that they actually work.
astringents	zinc oxide, calamine, hamamelis water (witch hazel)	"Tighten up" the skin and external tissue. May relieve irritation. Avoid tannic-acid-containing agents.
counterirritant	menthol	Menthol is the only FDA-approved agent here.
keratolytics	aluminum chlorhydroxy allantoinate	Causes surface skin cells to loosen and slough off. Of doubtful value. Must never be used on mucous membranes.
"wound healers," antiseptics, anticholinergics	No safe and effective agents exist.	There is no sound evidence that wound healers are safe and effective despite the continued sale of shark liver oil, cod liver oil, live yeast cell derivatives, and Peruvian balsam.

Misuse potential: high

Adverse effects: Self-medication with products containing benzocaine has been known to lead to allergic reactions. Vaso-constrictors such as epinephrine can conceivably enter the general circulation, where they could affect heart rate and blood pressure, or possibly worsen diabetes or hyperthyroidism.

Drug interactions: If you use a vasoconstrictor product, do not concurrently take any monoamine oxidase inhibitor such as Parnate or Nardil, as a dangerous increase in blood pressure could occur.

See also COUNTERIRRITANTS, LOCAL ANESTHETICS, PRAMOXINE, PREPARATION H

Heroin

Other name: diacetylmorphine
Source: chemical acetylation of morphine
Pharmacology: narcotic analgesic, antitussive, but not legal in United States
Dose: Heroin is not legal for any use in the United States

Heroin (diacetylmorphine) does not occur as such in nature. It was first prepared in Germany in 1874 by acetylation of the two hydroxyl groups in morphine (heroin comes from the German word *Heroisch*—they thought it was a *very* effective drug). Heroin thus exemplifies the partially synthetic or modified naturally occurring type of drug. Heroin was introduced into medicine in 1898 by Dr. Heinrich Dreser of the Bayer Company as a cough suppressant (antitussive) and pain reliever (analgesic). Dreser touted heroin as a safe, nonaddictive substitute for morphine. For years the medical profession remained ignorant of its potential for inducing physical dependence. In fact, it took 12 years and millions of addicted patients before doctors realized what we know today: Heroin is one of the most dangerous of the addicting drugs.

Pure heroin base is a white solid with a bitter taste; it melts at 173°C. Heroin hydrochloride melts at 243–44°C. Street heroin may be brown in color due to impurities not removed during its manufacture, or to the presence of a diluent (diluting agent used to "cut" it) such as cocoa or brown sugar. Eastern U.S. street heroin is different from the western preparation, even though both may be brown. While the western variety is usually cut with procaine (a local anesthetic), eastern heroin usually contains quinine. Talc, flour, and cornstarch have been used to dilute heroin, and there have been numerous cases of addicts with talc and cornstarch emboli (clots) in their lungs and eyes. This embolism is the result of direct injection of the heroin and its insoluble diluents into the bloodstream. In recent years the average purity of street heroin has been 5%, according to the DEA.

As a chemical substance, heroin begins in a clandestine laboratory, where the crude opium of illicit traffic is extracted and its morphine content isolated. An acetylating agent such as acetic anhydride is used to convert the morphine to diacetylmorphine (heroin).

Possession, sale, transport, and distribution of heroin are totally banned in the United States. The only heroin here is the illicit stuff on the streets. In England, sale and use of heroin is still legal, although very little of it is actually dispensed.

Heroin is a powerful narcotic analgesic and cough suppressant. It acts on the same body receptors as all the other opiates and is one of the most persuasively addicting substances known. ("It's so good, don't even try it once.") The DEA says there are about 500,000 heroin addicts in the United States, but there probably are more. Addicts in the United States spend about $10 billion a year to buy their heroin.

Heroin, although highly addictive and outlawed, is an excellent pain reliever, long considered by some to be more effective than morphine. It is available in 30 countries for use in pain relief and research, but not in the United States. A bill proposing the legalization of heroin for treatment of pain from cancer has been introduced in Congress by proponents who claim that heroin is more effective than morphine and can be given in smaller doses. However, in a recent study reported in the *New England Journal of Medicine,* Dr. C. E. Inturrisi of the Memorial Sloan-Kettering Cancer Center said, "The rationale in believing heroin itself does something morphine does not do becomes less and less likely when you consider [that] heroin must be converted into morphine first." Inturrisi found that before heroin can relieve pain, it must be chemically broken down into morphine and another chemical called 6-acetyemorphine. In a double-blind test, heroin addicts could not distinguish between heroin and morphine. This study seems to show that heroin is not a more effective analgesic than morphine.

Heroin does, however, pass the blood-brain barrier faster than morphine, thus giving a more acutely pleasureful rush than morphine.

Heroin overdosage, a frequent occurrence in the drug culture, can kill by respiratory depression. Naloxone (Narcan) is a narcotic antagonist that has found important use in emergency rooms for reversing the respiratory depression produced by heroin overdosage. Narcan is so effective in reversing heroin's effects that its use can actually precipitate a withdrawal syndrome in the addict.

Since 1964 heroin addiction has been treated with, among other approaches, methadone maintenance. See the section on methadone.

Abuse potential: high

Adverse effects: Heroin is not a chronically toxic drug in the human. Many addicts take large, daily doses for years and the worst they suffer is "nodding off" right after the hit, pinpoint pupils, or constipation. Heroin addicts function quite well in a variety of jobs. However, the addiction potential for heroin is exceedingly high; the serious user is very likely going to become an addict. He or she will develop a prodigious tolerance for the drug with a desire to reexperience its euphoric effects over and over again. Once physically addicted, the user will find it very difficult to stop taking the drug, and if he or she tries, the withdrawal syndrome is physically very hard to get through. Serious users of heroin are always in danger of overdosing on an unexpectedly potent batch, with consequent depression of respiration. If enough heroin is taken, respiration can stop altogether. Some others may die of anaphylactic shock from impurities in the heroin sample.

Drug interactions: Combining heroin with other brain depressants such as tranquilizers or antihistamines can lead to oversedation. The concurrent use of narcotics and monoamine oxidase inhibitors such as Parnate or Nardil may lead to a dangerous excitation of the brain with changes in blood pressure.

See also MORPHINE, NARCOTIC ANALGESICS, OPIATES, TOLERANCE, WITHDRAWAL SYNDROME

I

Icy Hot Balm. *See* COUNTERIRRITANTS

Isoamyl Nitrite. *See* NITRITES

Isotretinoin

Other name: Accutane
Source: synthesis
Pharmacology: acne drug
Dose: For acne, 0.5–2.0 mg/kg of body weight given in 2 divided doses daily for 15–20 weeks (most patients will benefit from 0.5–1.0 mg/kg/per day, and many will not require the full 15–20 weeks of therapy.) After a period of 2 months off the drug, a second regimen may be started.

Isotretinoin, hailed as a great advance in the treatment of acne, is discussed fully in the section on acne drugs. Because it is so effective and widely accepted by practitioner and patient, certain cautions regarding this drug bear repeating here. CAUTION: Women who are pregnant or even suspect that they might be pregnant must avoid this drug at all costs. Use an effective form of contraception for at least one month after the last dose of drug has been taken. Accutane is classified in pregnancy category X (see the section on pregnancy categories). It has been established that isotretinoin is powerfully capable of causing birth defects.

Misuse potential: medium. The danger lies in the teratogenic effects.

Adverse effects: Users of this drug can expect some dryness of the mouth and nose, lip inflammation, and dryness of the skin with itching. There have been instances of skin infections, exacerbation of arthritis, corneal eye damage, interference with normal red and white blood cell synthesis, headache, nausea, and vomiting associated with the use of isotretinoin. CAUTION: There is a statistical relationship between the use of Accutane and the occurrence of benign intracranial hypertension. If you experience headache, nausea, vomiting, or visual disturbances while taking this drug, report them to your physician immediately. Diabetics may have problems with blood sugar control and should have blood glucose levels checked frequently during treatment with this drug.

Drug interactions: Do not take any form of vitamin A concurrently with isotretinoin because of a possible increase in blood level of cholesterol.

See also ACNE DRUGS

J

Jimsonweed

Other names: Datura stramonium, devil's apple, stinkweed, thorn apple

Source: plant

Pharmacology: hallucinogen and hypnotic

Dose: The plant is not used in medicine.

Named after Jamestown, Virginia, jimsonweed is a plant member of the *Datura* genus. It is grown as an ornamental in many areas of the United States, and probably few people realize that it contains some very potent, potentially dangerous ingredients. At least one 20-year-old youth didn't. Anticipating a hallucinogenic experience, he made a drink by blending orange juice with jimsonweed, drank a large dose, and died in a hospital. Many species of the *Datura* genus are known; all produce long, trumpet-shaped flowers.

The 2 most important active ingredients in *Datura* are atropine and scopolamine (they are found in other plants, too, including belladonna). These 2 tropane alkaloids inhibit the action of acetylcholine. Thus they cause dry mucous membranes, dilated pupils, fever, and a too-fast heart rate. In large doses they can cause hallucinations, muscular incoordination, restlessness, and delirium. In very large doses the blood pressure falls dangerously, circulatory collapse occurs, and death from respiratory failure is possible. We are dealing here with very potent drugs having strong effects in milligram doses.

Stramonium products have been sold OTC to treat asthma; OTC scopolamine sleep aids still are available. Both can cause poisoning from an accidental or deliberate overdose in anticipation of a hallucinogenic experience. Children are especially vulnerable to the effects of atropine and scopolamine.

Abuse potential: high

Adverse effects: The most dangerous drug in Jimsonweed is atropine, with scopolamine a close second. While small doses of atropine slow the heart, doses of 2–10 mg cause very rapid heart rates, plus hot, dry, flushed skin; restlessness; excitement; and hallucinations. The delirium and coma that occur from very large doses can cause death. Atropine's effects in the human are mostly predictable, but idiosyncratic responses to scopolamine are common. Both atropine and scopolamine cause dryness of the mouth, difficulty in talking, and blurred vision. Of course, no one can predict how much atropine or scopolamine are contained in the jimsonweed concoctions made by the thrill seeker.

Drug interactions: Phenothiazine antipsychotics such as Thorazine, Vesprin, and Compazine can increase the effects of atropine, as can the antipsychotic drugs Prolixin and Permitil. Monoamine oxidase inhibitors such as Parnate and Nardil can increase the effects of atropine.

See also ATROPINE, HALLUCINOGENS

Jojoba

Other name: none
Source: plant (wild or cultivated)
Pharmacology: purported cure-all
Dose: applied externally

Jojoba oil, prepared from the jojoba bean, has been popular in the United States since its introduction in 1975. The plant grows wild in the deserts of Mexico and also is cultivated for its oil, which is quite expensive.

Jojoba oil has been touted as a treatment for many ills, but mostly as a treatment for teenage acne, dry skin, and for thinning hair. It is found in a popular, expensive shampoo.

Many people believe that jojoba is a great substance, but there is no scientific evidence to support it. The reports are anecdotal and the ads for it are hardly objective. The molecular structure of jojoba oil is distinctly different from that of the usual vegetable oil, but the importance of that information remains in doubt. The reports that it helps prevent thinning of hair or actually promotes hair growth are highly suspicious; if it really did that, it would sell like hotcakes.

Until we have some hard, objective facts on jojoba oil, we can regard it only as another interesting vegetable oil that makes a useful but expensive shampoo.

K

Kaopectate

The name Kaopectate comes from the two ingredients, kaolin and pectin. Although the name is catchy, the results are not, for the FDA has concluded that Kaopectate fails to show evidence of effectiveness for the use intended.

When Kaopectate was matched against a placebo (see the section on placebos), it failed to produce better results. It pays to remember that most (but not all) acute diarrheal attacks we experience are self-limiting and will clear up by themselves without the use of any chemical agent. (If the diarrhea occurs with a high fever or lasts more than 2 days, consult a physician.)

See also DIARRHEA PRODUCTS

Krebiozen. *See* QUACKERY

L

Laetrile. *See* QUACKERY

Laughing Gas. *See* NITROUS OXIDE

Laxatives

Americans are a super-bowel-conscious society. We spend over $300 million yearly on the purchase of more than 700 OTC laxative products. Apparently we believe the ads that suggest we must be regular if we are to be healthy and happy and that one day without a bowel movement is tantamount to chronic constipation. Well, there is a true story, documented, of a man who did not have a bowel movement for one whole year and who lived to tell about it. The truth is that many healthy people defecate promptly whenever they feel the urge, without resorting to a rigid, daily schedule. Furthermore, our eating habits and diet can change from day to day, and the presence or absence of bulk (cellulose), bran, prunes, or other foods can influence emptying of the colon. Degree of body hydration is reflected in stool consistency. Astronauts spending time in space travel know that a diet can be followed that leaves practically no residue.

In actual fact, then, normal elimination may be anywhere from twice daily to twice weekly. However, it is difficult to convince some people of this. Through family training or by association with health faddists, they have come to believe that daily defecation is very important if "toxic wastes" are to be eliminated. Thus they resort to laxatives (or daily enemas). These individuals are especially receptive to advertising that suggests that their sluggishness is due to their "sluggish" bowels. They fall for the baloney that they need to use a "colon cleanser." What they may fail to perceive is that left alone, the healthy rectum will take care of itself, and the more we stimulate it artificially to produce, the less likely it will do so on its own.

Other individuals do indeed suffer from chronic constipation, and they benefit from laxative administration. Genuine constipation may be tied to emotional stress, may be postsurgical, or may be due to a serious disease such as cancer. Antacid drugs can induce constipation, as can the opioid narcotics and certain antispasmodics.

In the following table, laxatives are classified on their basis of action:

Basis of Action	Laxative Examples
fecal softeners	mineral oil, dioctyl sodium sulfosuccinate, dioctyl calcium sulfosuccinate
saline cathartics	Epsom salt (magnesium sulfate), milk of magnesia (magnesium hydroxide), magnesium citrate
bulk formers	psyllium seed, methylcellulose, sodium carboxymethylcellulose, gums (for example, tragacanth), brans
stimulant (contact) cathartics	bisacodyl, phenophthalein, castor oil cascara, senna

Fecal softeners are just that, agents that mix with the feces and soften them so that elimination is easier. Mineral oil is not well absorbed from the GI tract and this can act as a fecal softener. It suffers from the serious disadvantage of being capable of dissolving fat-soluble vitamins such as A, D, E, and K, which are then excreted with the feces. For this reason, mineral oil is to be condemned as a laxative, especially if it is used repeatedly. Colace, a stool softener of the dioctyl sodium sulfosuccinate type, is actually a surfactant that is promoted for use in cardiac and other patients who must avoid difficult or painful defecation. In Peri-Colace, a stimulant cathartic has been added to the product.

Saline cathartics work because they remain inside the intestine and attract large volumes of water from the surrounding tissues. The water acts to soften the stool, promote peristalsis, and hasten the emptying of the bowel. Magnesium sulfate (Epsom salts) is the most well-known saline cathartic.

Bulk-forming laxatives act through their ability to absorb water and swell to a large, soft bolus of material inside the lumen of the intestine. This action promotes peristalsis and maintains the feces in a hydrated, soft condition. Defecation is thereby promoted. It seems clear that Americans should include more natural bulk-forming foods in their diet: bran, vegetables, cereals, fresh fruits, celery. These foods contain a high percentage of cellulose, the nondigestible polysaccharide that is so abundant in nature and that has been called nature's laxative. It is even more clear that popular refined types of foods (sugar, white bread, white rice, cakes, ice cream) offer calories but little or no bulk and should not comprise our main dietary intake.

Phenolphthalein is an example of a contact (stimulant) cathartic and is used in a popular OTC chewing gum laxative. Castor oil and cascara sagrada are additional stimulant cathartics. They probably work by their irritant actions on the lining of the intestine and are to be considered the harshest of the various cathartic types. Painful cramping is a possible side effect in the use of contact cathartics.

The experts who deal with constipation problems, real or imagined, have some words of advice: Don't be anxious about bowel movements; don't promote anxiety in children about regularity; use laxatives as a last resort, and then only infrequently; eat wisely and allow regularity to take care of itself; haste does not make waste. And ignore the unconscionable ads that implore you to make a laxative your "friend" or a "member of the family."

Misuse potential: medium. Be aware that the more you depend on laxatives, the more dependent upon them you may become. The laxative habit is a bad habit because it turns a normal body process into an artificially stimulated one, and you may be helpless to do anything about it. Insidious advertising contributes greatly to this bad situation; it is to be condemned.

Adverse effects: Mineral oil, used as a fecal softener, can cause loss of fat-soluble vitamins from the gastrointestinal tract.

There is the possibility that some persons will be allergic to the psyllium seed powder that makes up Metamucil; if you are an asthmatic, see your doctor before taking or handling Metamucil. Chronic use of any laxative other than stool softeners may cause a depletion of fluid or potassium ion from the body, resulting in muscle weakness. The continued use of the powerful stimulant cathartics such as bisacodyl, senna, castor oil, and cascara can in time alter the lining and the muscle tone of the bowel or cause fissures of the anus or hemorrhoids. Use of milk of magnesia as a laxative, especially for days or weeks at a time, may cause alkalinization of the body, with consequent interference with digestion or the occurrence of kidney stones in susceptible persons. Patients with kidney disease should consult their physician before using products containing magnesium.

Drug interactions: Laxatives speed up the movement of intestinal contents; this may result in decreased absorption of oral anticoagulants or vitamin K. Magnesium hydroxide is well known for its ability to bind drugs to its surface. That means that if you take it concurrently with a prescription drug, there is the possibility that the prescription drug will attach itself to the magnesium hydroxide, be excreted, and never do you any good. Drugs that bind to magnesium hydroxide include indomethacin (Indocin), chlorpromazine, and digitalis. Other drugs can bind, too, and you should consult your physician before concurrent use of milk of magnesia and any prescription drug. Magnesium ion (along with calcium and aluminum) may diminish the absorption of tetracycline antibiotics. You can eliminate this interaction by spacing the doses 2–3 hours apart. Magnesium salts can potentiate the neuromuscular blocking actions of muscle relaxants such as succinylcholine, tubocurarine, and decamethonium. Vitamin D products may promote increased absorption of magnesium; in kidney failure patients this could cause problems of magnesium toxicity.

See also CARTER'S LITTLE PILLS

Lobeline. *See* BANTRON SMOKING DETERRENT

Locker Room. *See* NITRITES

Look-alikes

A look-alike is a sly replica of a famous, legitimate pharmaceutical drug and designed to look exactly like a controlled substance but be perfectly legal because it actually contains only legal, salable OTC drugs. Over 100 mail order counterfeit products have been available that look just like amphetamines, Quaalude, and CNS depressants and stimulants. Cocaine look-alikes are legion: CocoSnow, Toot, Pseudocaine, Milky Trails, Florida Snow, Speckled Pups. Look-alike tablets and capsules are made in the same color, size, and shape as the real drug, and often with an imprinted identifying name or number that closely resembles that of the real prescription drug.

Central nervous system stimulant look-alikes typically contain caffeine (100–200 mg), ephedrine (12–25 mg), and phenylpropanolamine (35–50 mg), a combination that can pack quite a wallop! In addition, cocaine look-alikes may contain benzocaine, an OTC local anesthetic that simulates cocaine's anesthetic action. Sedative look-alikes contain 25–50 mg of the antihistamine doxylamine, the same drug found in the proprietaries Formula 44 and NyQuil. Phenylpropanolamine is the active ingredient in many OTC weight-loss pills that act by suppressing appetite.

Look-alikes are advertised nationally, often in student newspapers. They have been offered free to youngsters with the advice that they are "100% legal" and not as potent or as dangerous as the real thing. Nevertheless, poisonings and deaths have resulted, as in the dozen fatalities from the use of replica "black beauties" that looked just like the real Biphetamines.

Until recently, all look-alike products were legal. Now, however, 30 states have enacted look-alike substance acts, and the federal government has banned the OTC sale of stimulant products containing any active ingredient other than caffeine. This still leaves some loopholes for the sale of other look-alike products.

Abuse potential: high
Adverse effects: Stimulant look-alikes already contain heavy

doses of drugs that excite the brain and heart. Sensitive persons are going to suffer from insomnia, too-rapid heart rate, and general hyperexcitation. In addition, if the user engages in very strenuous activity, he or she will add epinephrine and other natural body stimulants to the drugs already present. A very excited state could result in which blood pressure rises dangerously and the heart is considerably taxed.

Conversely, sedative look-alikes contain large doses of brain depressants. If a person takes a legitimate antihistamine or sleep aid after having ingested the look-alike, serious depression of the brain could occur; driving a car or operating machinery could be hazardous.

Probably the biggest risk for the drug user is underestimating the strength of the drugs used in the look-alike product. If just 3 stimulant pills (see the second paragraph of this section) were taken, the total dose would be as much as 600 mg of caffeine (equivalent to 5–6 cups of freshly brewed coffee), 75 mg of ephedrine (capable of causing throbbing headache, tremor, and heart palpitations), and 150 mg of phenylpropanolamine (capable of causing high blood pressure and brain seizures, if we believe some authorities).

Drug interactions: Stimulant look-alikes when combined with caffeine from beverages can cause excessive stimulation of the brain. The same is true for amphetamine combinations. Sedative look-alikes when combined with antihistamines, tranquilizers, narcotic painkillers, or barbiturates can cause dangerous oversedation.

See also CAFFEINE, DOXYLAMINE, EPHEDRINE, PHENYL-PROPANOLAMINE

LSD

Other names: LSD-25, lysergic acid diethylamide
Source: partial synthesis
Pharmacology: hallucinogen
Dose: 50–150 micrograms (one-five-millionth of a pound); not used therapeutically

In 1938, Albert Hofmann, working for the Sandoz Company in Switzerland, synthesized a chemical that had never appeared on the face of the earth. He took lysergic acid, obtained as a chemical portion of the ergot alkaloids, and made the diethylamide derivative. The result was lysergic acid diethylamide, now known throughout the world as the hallucinogen LSD. The new compound was examined in the usual pharmacological screens and was placed "on the shelf."

Five years later, on April 16, 1943, Hofmann again had an opportunity to handle lysergic acid diethylamide. Ordinary manipulation of the substance was sufficient to cause accidental ingestion (probably through the skin), and the world's first LSD trip became history. Although not fully understanding what was happening, scientist Hofmann took careful note of his mental and physical reactions, as he also did several days later after he deliberately took a large dose of the drug. He experienced an intoxicated-like state in which his field of vision was greatly distorted. Colorful, plastic, fantastic images passed before his closed eyes. Everything was drenched in changing colors, predominantly disagreeable greens and blues. Sounds became translated into optical sensations, kaleidoscopically changing in form and color. Physically he noted a metallic taste on the tongue; dry and constricted throat; and arms and legs heavy, as if filled with lead. Alternately stupefied, then again clearly aware of the situation, he noted as though he were a neutral observer—standing outside of himself—that he shouted half crazily or talked unintelligibly.

LSD's psychotomimetic effects (mimicking a psychosis) were published in 1947, and it was revealed that the substance was psychoactive in exceedingly small amounts. As little as 100 micrograms (one-ten-thousandth of a gram or one-five-millionth of a pound) would suffice to turn a healthy adult into a basket case, at least temporarily. On a weight basis, LSD as a hallucinogen is some 5000–10,000 times more active than mescaline.

By 1949, LSD was being investigated in Europe and in the United States for possible therapeutic use in alcoholics, the mentally ill, and the sexually maladjusted. It was given to artists to see if they would become more creative, and to many other people and animals in many situations. In none of these applications did LSD emerge as a useful drug. It was discovered that LSD produced dilated pupils, a flushed face, a rise in body temperature, an increase in heart rate, goose bumps, salivation, perspiration, rapid development of tolerance, no addiction, but cross-tolerance to mescaline and psilocybin. "Flashbacks" were noted in which the hallucinogenic effects of the drugs were experienced weeks or months after use of the drug was completely discontinued.

The mythologization and criminalization of LSD in the 1960s and its subsequent classification as a Schedule I drug of high abuse potential are closely connected with the story of Timothy Leary, a Harvard professor until his dismissal in 1963. In 1966, all legal distribution of LSD in the United States was stopped, and today the only source of the drug for laypeople is the street. LSD is distributed in tablet form or in solution, absorbed into a sugar cube or almost any porous, absorbable substance. Since the usual dose of about 50–100 micrograms is too small a quantity to weigh out, the drug is always found diluted in some other substance. For example, LSD has been found in candy, paper ("blotter acid"), thin squares of gelatin ("window pane acid"), aspirin, jewelry, liquor, cloth, and even on the back of postage stamps. Obviously it is very easy to transport large numbers of doses of LSD, and detection is very difficult.

Just how LSD acts to produce hallucinations and altered perception remains in doubt. Research has shown that serotonin (5-hydroxytryptamine) is somehow involved. There is evidence that serotonin receptors in the brain are blocked or modified by LSD. Successful treatment of a bad LSD trip can often be accomplished in a conservative manner by friends of the user who "talk him or her down" in familiar surroundings. Minor tranquilizers or barbiturates, taken by injection, have proved useful, but the use of an antipsychotic drug (major tranquilizer) should be restricted to serious episodes of prolonged psychotic behavior.

An LSD trip can last 10–12 hours. Most of the dose is metabolized in the liver, and no more than 10% is eliminated from the body unchanged. Because tolerance to the effects of LSD develops very quickly, it cannot be used continually. As few as three daily doses can induce tolerance, and three or more days of abstinence may be required to overcome it. Tolerance does not develop with occasional use.

LSD remains high on the Drug Enforcement Administration's list of drugs to be controlled (it is a Schedule I drug). Its availability appears to be on the increase again, with illegal synthesis and sales apparently concentrated in the western United States, specifically in the San Francisco Bay area. It is suspected that LSD chemists, formerly in prison but now free, may be back at their illicit operations. In the NIDA Statistical Series for 1982 (DAWN data), LSD appears in twenty-ninth place (1.25%) of all drugs mentioned most frequently in hospital emergency rooms.

Abuse potential: high

Adverse effects: Many tens of thousands of hallucinogenic "trips" have been taken over the past 30 years, most under the influence of LSD. Early on it was noted that in certain sensitive people psychotic breaks could be precipitated by the hallucinogen. In others, the experience was termed a "bummer"—that is, there were unpleasant, disturbing, even psychotic episodes that made the person believe he or she was losing their mind. LSD also produces physical effects: dilated pupil, flushed face, chilliness, a rise in body temperature, an increase in heart rate, goose bumps, salivation, and perspiration. In the long term, LSD is well known for producing flashbacks in a small percentage of users. In this phenomenon the user spontaneously reexperiences LSD-like symptoms weeks or months after the last dose was taken. There is no way to stop the flashback, which may involve considerable dread and panic. People do not become physically dependent on LSD but can become psychologically dependent on it.

Drug interactions: Concurrent use of epinephrine, dopamine, or brain stimulants such as the amphetamines or hallucinogenic amphetamine derivatives can induce a dangerous psychotic state.

See also HALLUCINOGENS, PSYCHEDELICS

M

Maalox. *See* ANTACIDS

Magaldrate

Other name: Riopan
Source: compounding
Pharmacology: antacid
Dose: Between meals and at bedtime: 1–2 teaspoonfuls of suspension, or 1–2 tablets (approximately 0.5–1.0 g). Take with adequate water.

Although acid in the stomach is normal, healthy, and necessary for proper digestion, there are times when it is beneficial to neutralize excess stomach acid chemically. Peptic ulcer, inflammation of the esophagus and stomach, and hiatal hernia are all made worse by the presence of excessive acid.

A great number and variety of antacids are available OTC for self-medication or use under a doctor's supervision (see the section on antacids). Magaldrate is one of the antacids that contain both magnesium and aluminum hydroxides, but it is unique in that it is a chemical entity, not the usual physical mixture. It has a lower neutralizing capacity than a physical mixture, but the manufacturer contends that it shows a buffering effect as well as a neutralizing effect.

Riopan is promoted for symptomatic relief of heartburn, "sour" stomach, acid indigestion, and upset stomach. Note that all of these are vague terms for uncertain conditions. An antacid can help relieve symptoms, but it would be far wiser to get at the reason behind the symptoms. Is it an offending food, job stress, overeating, or alcohol consumption?

Misuse potential: medium

Adverse effects: It is all too easy to listen to the misleading ads and overrely on an antacid. Overreliance leads to habituation and compulsive use. This is dangerous because antacids can change the normal acid-base balance of our body, possibly leading to kidney stones in susceptible people. Unless your doctor can find a medical reason for taking an antacid, you are far better off not taking them.

CAUTION: FOLLOW LABEL DIRECTIONS. Do not take more than 20 teaspoonfuls (or tablets) in any 24-hour period. If you suffer from kidney disease, see a doctor before taking any antacid. As with any suspension, shake the bottle well before using.

CAUTION: With prolonged use, Riopan can cause a dangerous loss of body phosphorus.

Drug interactions: There are two ways antacids can interfere with other drugs: by changing gastrointestinal (GI) absorption, and by affecting kidney elimination. Antacids of the aluminum, calcium, and magnesium type can bind to (or absorb) many prescription drugs, thus decreasing their absorption from the GI tract. Examples of drugs that can be bound are: tetracycline antibiotics, digitalis drugs, indomethacin, and chlorpromazine. Consult your physician before concurrent use of any prescription drug and an antacid. Proper spacing of doses of antacids and prescription drugs can eliminate possible interactions. Because antacids tend to make the GI tract alkaline, they can cause enteric-coated tablets to dissolve faster.

See also ANTACIDS

Magnesium Hydroxide. *See* ANTACIDS, LAXATIVES

Marijuana

Other names: known as or represented by angel dust, cannabis, charas, ganja, hashish, hash oil, pot, sinsemilla, THC, Thai sticks

Sources: the plant *Cannabis sativa* and other species

Pharmacology: sedative, tranquilizer, mild hallucinogen

Dose: The intake of 5–10 mg (an average marijuana joint) of THC into the bloodstream is sufficient to get "high."

Cannabis is a tall annual weed, sometimes reaching a height of 4 meters (13 feet). The male and female plants grow in almost any waste or fertile area. Scientific cultivation of cannabis plants has revealed remarkable variations in plant characteristics, size, and concentration of active ingredients. It is not clear whether cannabis is a single genus composed of more than 100 species or a single species that has many variations. Plant scientists recognize the Indian, Mexican, Thai, Korean, Iowan, and Russian variants, differing as much as fiftyfold in their tetrahydrocannabinol concentration (0.07–3.7%). The predominant, wild-growing U.S. form of marijuana is *C. sativa,* cultivated on great plantations in early America for its hemp fiber, used in rope and cloth. Hemp seeds are rich in oil and have long been used throughout the world as a source of food. As a medicine, marijuana was important not only to peoples of ancient China and India but also to physicians in Europe and the United States in the late 1800s and early 1900s. Marijuana was official in the *USP* in the early 1930s; a fluid extract was sold as a treatment for neuralgia, mental depression, rheumatism, and gout.

Concurrent with licit uses through the centuries was the illicit consumption of marijuana for its euphoriant and intoxicant effects. Chemists have identified 421 different compounds in marijuana; the heat produced by smoking causes chemical changes that increase this number to over 2000. There are 61 different fat-soluble cannabinoids in marijuana, and 11 of these are specifically termed tetrahydrocannabinols. The major active euphoric ingredient is delta-9-tetrahydrocannabinol (THC). (The distinction between delta-9-THC and delta-8-THC is based on the position of the carbon-to-carbon double bond in the THC molecule; a newer system of numbering designates delta-9 as delta-1-THC.)

In *hashish,* the compressed, resinous mixture made from the flowering tops of female cannabis plants, the concentration of THC is 10–20%. Historically, "hasheesh" has been smoked, eaten, or drunk by millions of people, especially in Moslem areas of North Africa and the Near East. *Hash oil,* from the oily resin on the leaves, contains 30–40% THC. There is less THC in cannabis leaves and practically none in the stems, roots, or seeds. Somewhat less potent preparations are *bhang* and *ganja.* The term *sinsemilla* (meaning "without seeds") refers to the product made from specially cultivated flowering tops of unfertilized female plants. Much sinsemilla is grown illicitly in California and is prized for its high THC content (up to 8%). *Thai sticks* (from Thailand) are 6-to-12-inch-long compressed bundles of buds and stems of high THC content. The "sticks" are the form in which the drug is transported; for use, the bundles are broken up and smoked as a joint (cigarette) or in pipes. Angel dust is a mixture of mint leaves, parsley, or low-grade marijuana laced with PCP.

Officially, all of these preparations are grouped together under the term *cannabis.* The "pot" or "grass" available to most American users today is of increasingly higher THC concentration. In the 1960s THC averaged 0.1–2%; in the 1970s it averaged 1%; today it averages 2–5%. In smoking a typical joint, the user will receive a dose of 5–25 mg of THC, assuming that he or she is smoking one of the more potent batches. With more than 20 million Americans using it daily, pot is the most widely used drug in the nation.

In 1937, with the passage of the Marijuana Tax Act, marijuana became an outlaw drug. In that same year, all 48 states and the District of Columbia had antimarijuana laws in their codes. Our latest law on the subject, the 1970 Controlled Substances Act, classifies pot as a high-abuse-potential drug with no medical value and places it in Schedule I (in spite of which, the drug *is* used medicinally; see later in this section).

Since the 1970s, authorities have sprayed the herbicide paraquat on fields of growing marijuana in attempts to destroy the plant at its source. Spraying with this herbicide is controversial because of the possible toxic effects of paraquat residues in the pot that gets to the illicit market. For this reason the National Organization for the Reform of Marijuana Laws (NORML) has filed lawsuits to delay spraying.

The intake of 5–10 mg of THC into the bloodstream is sufficient to get high (or "stoned"). A marijuana high is a combination of sedation, tranquilization, and mild hallucination. The user experiences mood changes involving mild euphoria; a relaxed, dreamy reverie; a feeling of well-being; heightened appreciation of sounds and colors; remembrance of pleasure, but perhaps also imperception of time and space; a lag between thought and reaction; less precise thinking; and a flattened affect. He or she may experience hunger, thirst, and uncontrollable laughter, or nausea, dizziness, and dryness of the mouth. Not all of these effects are experienced by every user. Infrequently, panic reactions are reported, with feelings of persecution, confusion, and fear. This seems to occur especially in the neophyte user taking high doses. In general, high doses of THC can cause illusions, pseudohallucinations, and paranoid thinking.

There is now general agreement that even moderate doses of pot can cause short-term memory loss, impaired intellectual functioning, and impaired ability to read with comprehension, to acquire, store, and recall information, and to communicate clearly. Attention span, tracking, and perception may be impaired. These reactions are all dose-related and temporary.

The cannabinols in pot cause dose-related tachycardia (faster-than-normal heart rate), increasing the rate to as high as 160 beats per minute. Long-term users develop a tolerance to this effect; there appears to be no damage to the healthy heart. Blood vessels in the eye are dilated, giving a bloodshot-eye effect. Ears become warm and red. Postural hypotension (dizziness upon standing) is seen.

In a moderate dose THC causes bronchodilation and might be useful in asthma, but heavy use has the opposite effect, causing slight obstruction of air passages. Those who smoke pot heavily experience inflammation of the bronchi, sore throat, and inflamed sinuses. Marijuana smoke has more tar than cigarette smoke (3 marijuana joints equal 20 tobacco cigarettes a day), and the practice of smoking the joint down to the end ensures that the tars get into the smoker's lungs. Pot smoke has as much polycyclic carcinogens as and more mutagens than tobacco smoke. Rodent skins painted with marijuana tars develop tumors just as they do with tobacco tars, but direct confirmation of the generation of human lung tumors by marijuana has not yet been made. Passive inhalation of pot smoke can result in detectable blood levels of THC. Nonpot smokers sitting in a closed room and passively inhaling pot smoke achieved urine levels of THC as high as 50–100 nanograms per ml.

Marijuana unquestionably impairs driving ability, even after ordinary social use, and this effect can last for as long as 10–12 hours. Pot can impair pilots even 24 hours after its use. Experienced pilots who smoked 1 joint (containing 19 mg of THC) had trouble landing on a flight simulator 1 day after they smoked marijuana; 1 pilot missed the landing strip entirely.

Regarding actions and fate in the body, THC reaches the brain quickly and produces a euphoric high in 20–30 minutes. Its obvious effects disappear in 2–3 hours, but residual effects are demonstrable up to 10 hours after smoking a joint. THC is fat-soluble, and it and its breakdown products are stored in the brain, lungs, testes, ovaries, and body fat in general. Their slow release from these tissues permits their detection in the urine up to 10 days following the last dose. THC ingested by smoking or eating marijuana is biotransformed in the liver to 11-hydroxy-THC and then to 9-carboxy-THC. Also formed are 8-hydroxy-THC and 9,11-dihydroxy-THC. These compounds are referred to as metabolites of THC, and their detection in the body or urine is taken as definite proof of marijuana use. Chemistry laboratories are now equipped to detect THC and its metabolites in nanogram (billionths of a gram) quantities in the urine of pot smokers. One lab, using radioimmunoassay, can detect THC in the urine weeks after a single use. One study showed that because of its high fat solubility, THC in active form may be retained in the body for as long as 45 days after heavy smoking. See the section on testing for drugs for a discussion of false positive tests in marijuana detection.

Risks: The short-term risks to physical health in normal adults from occasional social smoking of marijuana appear to be minimal. Long-term smoking, especially in heavier amounts, can cause bronchitis, irritation of the respiratory tract, and significant abnormalities in lung tissue. While there is no proof, very-long-term inhalation of the mutagens and carcinogens in pot smoke very likely predisposes to cancer of the lung. Research reports on the effects of marijuana on reproduction are incomplete and sometimes contradictory, and because of this their significance is not clear. Pot appears to produce a brief fall in sperm production, and it alters sperm shape and mobility. In animals and probably in humans, THC reduces testosterone levels, but the significance of this finding remains in doubt. Pubescent boys appear to be especially at risk from a lowered testosterone level. Long-term administration of THC to mice caused an increase in abnormal ova (5.5% above those of the control group). Studies of women who used marijuana regularly during pregnancy showed that stillbirths and neonatal deaths increased. Three studies have implicated marijuana in a syndrome identical to the fetal alcohol syndrome. However, polydrug use in the women studied makes it difficult to pinpoint teratogenicity.

Preteenage boys; adults with marginal fertility; people with chronic heart disease, psychoses, or epilepsy; and pregnant and nursing women should not smoke pot, nor should people taking medicines for diabetes or epilepsy. Those who drive vehicles or operate machinery while under the influence of THC or its metabolites are at increased risk of accidents.

By 1978, 11 states had passed laws decriminalizing marijuana, but since then, none has. Decriminalization (not to be confused with legalization) means to ease the penalties for a still-illegal substance—that is, to consider the possession of small amounts of pot a misdemeanor (not a felony) and to reduce the fine to as little as $50 or even $5.00. It would appear that the attitude of the nation is again hardening against marijuana and that there is little chance of further reform in our marijuana laws.

Despite the fact that marijuana is a Schedule I controlled substance banned in all its aspects, it is extensively used in hundreds of hospitals across the nation to control the nausea and vomiting associated with chemotherapy for certain types of cancer. Special laws permit this to occur, and physicians annually treat some 8,000 to 10,000 patients with marijuana. In the disease called glaucoma, there is a dangerous increase in the pressure of the fluid inside the eyeball. It has been found that THC substantially reduces this pressure, generating proposals to use marijuana in treating glaucoma. For medical use, the Unimed Company has applied to the FDA to market THC capsules under the trade name Marinol.

Abuse potential: high

Adverse effects: Marijuana causes a rapid heart rate—up to 160 beats per minute—combined with dilated blood vessels in the eyes and ears. Users may experience dizziness upon standing. Heavy pot use causes inflammation of the throat, sinuses, and windpipes. The smoke from a marijuana cigarette contains cancer-causing chemicals, but proof of carcinogenicity in humans is lacking. Marijuana causes short-term memory loss and an unquestioned impairment of driving ability. There is a suspicion, but not clear proof, that pot causes the amotivational syndrome—that is, blunts enthusiasm, takes away drive, and leaves the user content to sit around all day, red-eyed but happy and hungry. In *burnout,* a term first used by marijuana smokers themselves, heavy use over very long periods makes the smoker dull, slow-moving, and so inattentive of surroundings that he or she fails to respond when spoken to and is completely unaware that a problem exists. Current concentrations of THC in marijuana are higher than ever, and more users are experiencing a marijuana freakout—that is, an acute anxiety attack something like the "bad trip" in an LSD experience. Marijuana greatly impairs tracking ability, the ability to follow a moving object such as a baseball.

Drug interactions: The combination of marijuana and tobacco smoke is worse than either alone in respect to damage to the lungs and bronchi. The concurrent use of alcohol and pot is especially effective in impairing driving skills and steadiness on the feet. Three drinks (1.5 fluid ounces of alcohol each) together with marijuana can cause intense nausea and vomiting. THC has a depressant effect upon the brain, and combining it with any other depressant such as a tranquilizer, barbiturate, antihistamine, or narcotic painkiller could lead to oversedation.

MDA. *See* HALLUCINOGENIC AMPHETAMINE
DERIVATIVES

MDM. *See* HALLUCINOGENIC AMPHETAMINE
DERIVATIVES

MDMA. *See* HALLUCINOGENIC AMPHETAMINE
DERIVATIVES

Menstrual Products

It may be difficult to distinguish between normal menstruation and dysmenorrhea (painful or difficult menstruation). In the latter there can be abnormal pain ranging from moderate to intense, accompanied by nausea, vomiting, and diarrhea. The pain may seem like colic or may be aching and may last from one hour to several days. Some women experience pelvic heaviness or breast fullness. A premenstrual syndrome (PMS) has now been defined and widely discussed.

Modern thought connects release of prostaglandins in the uterus with the discomfort of dysmenorrhea. Any drug that can block the synthesis of prostaglandins can relieve the symptoms (*see* aspirin).

Some of the menstrual products sold OTC are: Midol (discussed separately), Aqua-Ban, Odrinil, Premesyn PMS, Pursettes Premenstrual Tablets, Sunril Premenstrual Capsules, and Trendar Menstrual Relief Tablets. Some of these preparations contain nothing but diuretics for anticipated relief of bloating or fullness. CAUTION: Odrinil, a diuretic product containing buchu, uva ursi, corn silk, juniper, and caffeine, is discredited by the FDA as lacking evidence of safety and effectiveness. Lydia Pinkham's menstrual tablets likewise contain a hodge-podge of plant extracts (pleurisy root, licorice) and also are rejected by the FDA.

Most of the other menstrual products contain a painkiller such as acetaminophen, which is fine, but also an antihistamine or weak diuretic of questionable efficacy. Antihistamines do not relieve pain or aid in water loss and can cause problems because of their side effects.

Brand-name menstrual products are expensive. If you wish relief from pain, generic acetaminophen is an inexpensive alternative. If bloating is the problem, consuming less salt seven days prior to the menses could help.

Misuse potential: high

Adverse effects: Regarding acetaminophen-containing products, if you do not exceed the recommended label dose you probably will not experience any adverse effects. However, excessive doses of acetaminophen can cause damage to the liver and kidneys. CAUTION: Persons with a history of liver disease should consult their physician before using acetaminophen in extra-strength preparations or for long periods. The antihistamine contained in some products can cause drowsiness and impaired ability to drive a car or operate machinery.

Drug interactions: Acetaminophen can increase the effects of concurrently administered oral anticoagulants, conceivably leading to a bleeding tendency. Combining alcohol with acetaminophen can intensify the poisonous effects of both on the liver. Either avoid this drug combination or consult your doctor beforehand.

See also ACETAMINOPHEN, ANTIHISTAMINES, MIDOL

Meperidine. *See* DEMEROL

Meprobamate

Other names: Equanil, Miltown
Source: synthesis
Pharmacology: minor tranquilizer, muscle relaxant
Dose: Adults: The usual dosage is 1200–1600 mg daily in divided doses, not to exceed 2400 mg a day. Children: Ages 6–12 years, 100–200 mg 2–3 times a day. Not recommended for children under 6 years. Tablets typically contain 200 or 400 mg of meprobamate.

One important chemical type of minor tranquilizer is the propanediol carbamate, exemplified by the well-known prescription-only drugs Equanil and Miltown. These anxiety-reducing, muscle-relaxant drugs have been widely used to treat anxiety, muscle spasm, insomnia, *petit mal* epilepsy, and the symptoms of tetanus. They act much like the barbiturates, inducing sleep in large doses, suppressing REM sleep, and inducing the production of liver enzymes that hasten their own metabolism. They do *not* depress respiration nearly as much as the barbiturates, making it much more difficult to commit suicide using them. Meprobamates can also induce tolerance, physical dependence, and psychological dependence. At doses of 3200 mg a day (8 400-mg tablets) for a month, barbituratelike withdrawal symptoms can occur. These include convulsions, coma, and psychotic behavior.

Soma (carisoprodol) is a propanediol *di*carbamate that is promoted as a muscle relaxant to be used in conjunction with rest and physical therapy. Its use is contraindicated in pregnant women and children under 12 years.

Abuse potential: medium. Twenty-five years of experience has taught us that the danger with tranquilizers lies in our tendency to overrely on them, to use them longer than necessary, and too often to become dependent on them. Physical dependence with a serious withdrawal syndrome is a real possibility with the meprobamates. If you must use tranquilizers at all, use them only for a few days, or a week at most. Of course, if your doctor is closely supervising your use, that is another matter.

Adverse effects: Some users report drowsiness, dizziness, slurred speech, tingling in the extremities, nausea, vomiting, diarrhea, and allergic reactions that vary from itching and skin rash to fever and bronchospasm. Rarely have there been reports of damage to the blood-forming organs with consequent agranulocytosis. WARNING: Never use meprobamate during pregnancy, even for one day, because of the risk of birth defects. If you even think you might be pregnant, do not use this drug.

Drug interactions: Combining alcohol with meprobamate could result in oversedation of the brain, making the operation of a car or machinery dangerous. Meprobamate may interact to reduce the effectiveness of oral contraceptives, estrogens, and oral anticoagulants. Monoamine oxidase inhibitor drugs such as Parnate or Nardil combined with meprobamate may increase the brain-depressant action of the meprobamate.

See also TRANQUILIZERS, MINOR

Mescaline

Other names: active ingredient in peyote, peyotl, mescal button, cactus alkaloid

Source: the cactus *Lophophora williamsii*

Pharmacology: hallucinogen

Dose of abuse: 5 mg per kg body weight (about 2 mg per pound); not used in therapy; some 4–12 mescal buttons would supply a heavy dose for an average adult

Mescaline is the active hallucinogenic ingredient in the famous peyote cactus, found growing in the Rio Grande Valley, from Mexico City to the Texas border, and in some areas of Texas, Arizona, and California. The cactus is an unimpressive gray-green knob about the size of a golf ball but having a large taproot (which the DEA considers legally part of the peyote). Confusion has arisen over the term *peyote*, for it is used broadly and generally in Mexico for many species of cacti and other plants, not all of which are hallucinogenic.

Peyote was known to the Aztecs, who considered this hallucinogen a divine messenger. When used by natives in a religious ritual, the top of the cactus is sliced off, giving mescal "buttons," some 4–12 of which are ingested. A period of meditation follows, during which nausea and vomiting occur, accompanied by visual aberrations, sometimes of vast fields of gold jewels, changing kaleidoscopically. The natives feel removed from earthly cares. A peyote trip can last from 6–10 hours.

In the 1950s and 1960s mescaline was widely investigated as a possible therapeutic agent for epileptics, schizophrenics, and alcoholics. The idea was that this hallucinogen would provide the patient with insights into his or her disease and thus make a cure more likely. Mescaline also was used by artists who thought they might be able to increase their creativity. No important, broadly applicable uses were found. North American Indians comprising the Native American Church report that they have successfully used peyote in the treatment of widespread alcoholism.

Tolerance to the hallucinogenic effects of mescaline develops after repeated use, and this tolerance crosses over to LSD and psylocybin, which then also fail to produce hallucinations. Chemically, mescaline has a simple structure closely related to those of the amphetamines and not too far removed from those of the catecholamines. Mescaline owes its psychotropic activity to its effects upon nerves activated by norepinephrine.

Under the Controlled Substances Act, mescaline is a Schedule I drug; its mere possession, whether pure or as part of the cactus plant, is punishable. Mescal buttons can be found in the illegal drug trade, but mescaline itself is rarely encountered. According to the Do It Now Foundation, about 87% of the purported street samples of mescaline and mescal buttons are deceitful. Most are actually LSD or LSD-PCP mixtures.

Abuse potential: high

Adverse effects: Similar to the adverse effects caused by LSD and psylocybin, mescaline can cause an increase in heart rate and blood pressure, pupil dilation, a rise in body temperature, and a general stimulation of the brain. Psychologically speaking, mescaline is a powerful hallucinogen with the potential for psychological trauma. An adult male who took 1 mescal button (less than 25 mg of mescaline) was violently sick for 24 hours but did not hallucinate on this small dose. A 22-year-old female who received 400 mg of mescaline had an unpleasant paranoid reaction consisting of paranoia, impaired attention, and reduced emotional expression; for several days afterward she had auditory and visual hallucinations. A man who ingested 750 mg of pure mescaline suffered a severe psychotomimetic reaction that lasted for 16 hours; his haunting delusions and anxiety did not completely clear up until after 2 months.

Drug interactions: Since the brain is already stimulated by mescaline, concurrent use of epinephrine, dopamine, or brain stimulants such as the amphetamines or hallucinogenic amphetamine derivatives could induce a dangerous psychotic state.

See also HALLUCINOGENS, HALLUCINOGENIC AMPHETAMINE DERIVATIVES

Metabisulfite. *See* DRUG ALLERGIES

Metamucil

Other name of active ingredient: psyllium seed mucilage
Source: plant
Pharmacology: bulk-forming laxative
Dose: either 1 teaspoonful, 1 tablespoonful, or 1 packet, depending on preparation

This laxative belongs to the category of bulk formers, which means that the active ingredient swells up in contact with water in the bowel, and the resultant bulk promotes peristalsis and evacuation. This also helps keep the feces soft and more easily expelled.

Metamucil contains powdered psyllium seed, obtained from species of plantain (plantago seed). The seeds contain a natural mucilage that forms a gelatinous mass on contact with water. In Metamucil, the seeds are ground to a powder.

Other bulk formers used as laxatives are methylcellulose, carboxymethylcellulose sodium, tragacanth, and agar. Bran in the diet acts in much the same manner.

The makers of Metamucil offer it in various flavors, such as orange or strawberry, for customer acceptance, but one wonders if laxatives are *supposed* to taste delicious, or if they can be made so acceptable that the public is more likely to rely on them. Laxatives are unnatural. The normal person who includes a reasonable quantity of fiber in the diet and who drinks plenty of fluids will probably never need a laxative. However, elderly people or patients taking required medications may benefit from the use of bulk laxatives.

Misuse potential: medium

Adverse effects: Some people may be allergic to psyllium powder, either inhaled or taken internally. If you have a history of asthma or are allergic to drugs generally, consult with your physician before using this laxative. Falling prey to the laxative habit is a real possibility with this and any of the other laxative products. Healthy people who eat a variety of foods, including foods with a reasonable fiber content, will probably never have to resort to a laxative in their entire lifetime. If you give yourself time to defecate and get into the habit, you will not have to resort to artificial stimulation. But once you begin to rely seriously on a laxative, you may find yourself dependent upon it for what should be a natural act, and then you are hooked for possibly years. The laxative manufacturers, of course, want this to happen, and continue their barrage of advertising to ensure that it will happen. Ads have actually stated, "Make our product a member of your family," and "You will be regular for a lifetime." This is insidious advertising at its worst; don't fall for it.

Drug interactions: Metamucil can reduce the absorption of digoxin. There should be a two-hour interval between taking these drugs. There is some possibility that the increased speed of passage of intestinal contents, caused by laxatives, may result in a reduction of absorption of Vitamin K or oral anticoagulants. If this is a problem, the solution would be to stop using the laxative. Similarly, laxative-induced diarrhea could reduce the gastrointestinal absorption of isoniazid (INH, an antitubercular drug). Combining the anti-high-blood-pressure drug Inversine with a bulk-forming laxative could result in diminished absorption of the Inversine and loss of control of the high blood pressure.

See also LAXATIVES

Methadone

Other names: Adanon, Amidon, Dolophine
Source: synthesis
Pharmacology: narcotic analgesic
Dose: For analgesia, 2.5–10 mg. In detoxification, 15–20 mg usually will prevent opiate withdrawal symptoms. In maintenance, 40 mg a day are typical. Lilly's Dolophine is available in 5- and 10-mg tablets.

Developed in Germany in time for World War II, methadone has found wide use as a synthetic narcotic analgesic, an opioid, having nearly all the pharmacological activity of morphine. Methadone is an excellent painkiller in its own right, but most people recognize it as the key substance in American and British maintenance programs for the treatment of heroin addiction. Methadone itself is addictive.

Methadone detoxification and maintenance were pioneered in 1964 in New York City by Marie Nyswander and Vincent Dole. They conceived of the idea of opening a clinic and offering methadone and counseling to heroin addicts who expressed a desire to kick their addiction. Methadone does not give the pleasureful rush of heroin but it prevents heroin withdrawal symptoms, is cheap to make and administer, and its clinical use can be controlled. The detoxification *ideal,* then, is to get the heroin addict to substitute methadone for heroin and cooperate in reducing the dose a little each day until he or she is detoxified from all narcotics, gets a job, and reenters society. Unfortunately, too many addicts drop out of maintenance, fail to complete detoxification, secretly continue to use heroin, or sell their take-home weekend supply of methadone on the street. At best, a cure rate of 10–15% is all that can be expected from methadone maintenance. NOTE: If methadone is used in a heroin detoxification course, a time limit of 21 days is imposed. After that, the procedure passes from detoxification to maintenance, and maintenance is permitted by federal law to be conducted only in an approved methadone maintenance program.

It is also unfortunate that in New York City methadone itself has become a primary addictive drug, and clinics are admitting methadone addicts for first-time treatment.

In England, methadone has replaced heroin as the detoxification or maintenance drug for heroin addiction. Addicts are treated in hospitals and clinics, are given psychiatric and social counseling, and are given prescriptions for methadone.

Methadone acts on the central nervous system and on organs composed of smooth muscle. Methadone given by mouth is only about half as potent as when given by injection; it is available legally by prescription in the United States, and its effects last from 36 to 48 hours.

Abuse potential: high

Adverse effects: As any addict well knows, the adverse effects of methadone include constipation, sweating, insomnia, reduction of sexual drive, and inhibition of orgasm. Some users will experience flushing of the face, heart palpitations, dizziness, dry mouth, difficulty in urination, or possibly an allergic reaction manifested as skin rash, itching, redness, or edema. The major dangers from methadone overdosage are depression of respiration (serious enough at times to cause death) and depression of the heart and circulatory system. Shock and cardiac arrest have been seen in some users. Users must constantly be aware that methadone is an addicting narcotic drug, in the same category as morphine and heroin. Tolerance to it develops, and a withdrawal syndrome will be experienced upon abrupt withdrawal in the addict. The withdrawal is similar to that from morphine but develops more slowly, lasts longer, and is not so acutely difficult.

Drug interactions: Dilantin and Rifampin can speed up the body's metabolism of methadone, conceivably diminishing it to the point where withdrawal symptoms begin. Pentazocine (Talwin), another narcotic analgesic, when given concurrently also can start withdrawal symptoms because of its ability to act as a narcotic antagonist. Use of any brain-depressant drug such as alcohol, barbiturates, Dilantin, or tranquilizers in combination with methadone can be dangerous because of excessive depression of the brain, including respiratory depression.

See also NARCOTIC ANALGESICS

Methadone Maintenance. *See* METHADONE

Methamphetamine

Other names: Desoxyn, crank, crystal, crystal meth, Methedrine, splash, speed

Source: synthesis

Pharmacology: CNS stimulant, obesity control, sympathomimetic

Dose: For attention-deficit disorder with hyperactivity in children 6 years or older, an initial dose of 5 mg once or twice a day is usual, with a typical effective dose of 20–25 mg daily. Desoxyn tablets are supplied in the following strengths: 5 mg (white), 10 mg (orange), and 15 mg (yellow).

Under its trade name Desoxyn, methamphetamine has long been prescribed as an appetite suppressant in the treatment of obesity. However, Abbott Laboratories, the makers of Desoxyn, warns that it has not been established that the action of Desoxyn in treating obesity is primarily one of appetite suppression. Other actions on the brain or metabolism may be involved. Abbott also cautions that amphetamine use in weight control should be short-term (a few weeks or less) and restricted to patients who have failed to respond to diets or other programs. The reason for caution, of course, is that methamphetamine has a high potential for abuse. Its stimulant effect on the brain and its mood-altering potential can easily lead to tolerance and drug dependence. One 22-year-old housewife and would-be weight loser got hooked on Desoxyn and built her way up to 30 tablets a day.

In one study, housewives and other women who were either unemployed or retired were found to be among the highest regular users of amphetamine diet pills. Sales representatives also had high rates of use. Amphetamine use in "fat clinics" has gotten out of hand. The DEA has information on physicians who have ordered and received more than 3 million amphetamine dosage units in a year. A substantial amount of illegal diversion of stimulant drugs occurs through the operation of clinics devoted entirely to the treatment of obesity.

Taking "uppers" to lose weight is a bad idea from the start.

The side effects of nervousness and central excitation may cause users to resort to tranquilizers or sedatives to get to sleep. The next morning a bigger dose of stimulant may be needed to get going. And so on.

For all these reasons the FDA has recommended a ban on the use of any amphetamine in weight control; Wisconsin and Maryland have passed legislation that virtually assures such a ban. The FDA continues to approve use of amphetamines for narcolepsy and for hyperactivity in children.

A serious form of abuse involves individuals who find pleasure in the euphoric rush effects of injected amphetamine. The drug most often abused here is methamphetamine (the source of which is typically an illicit "crystal meth" lab located in somebody's garage or basement; literally hundreds of such labs have been raided in recent years). Called a speed freak, the user will mainline 20–40 mg of methamphetamine (speed) at first, then gradually increase the dose to hundreds of milligrams a day as tolerance develops. The user may go on an amphetamine spree, staying awake for days at a time, not wanting to come down off the euphoric high. He or she probably will eat nothing during the high and lose considerable weight. Then, exhausted and drained, the user will sleep for a day or more, awake hungry, and start the whole abusive process over again.

The speed freak is driven by a desire to reexperience the ecstasy of the high, which is described as being different from the high following an oral dose.

The possibility of a psychotic breakdown accompanies the heavy use of amphetamines, either from a single large dose or from chronic moderate doses. A paranoid psychosis may develop in which the individual believes that certain people are talking about the individual behind his or her back or that he or she is being followed everywhere. One user climbed to the roof of a building to escape secret agents and then threw tiles down on his imaginary pursuers. Auditory and visual hallucinations may accompany the psychosis, giving the impression that the speed freak is a schizophrenic. Heavy speed users can exhibit freakish, bizarre, and unpredictable behavior; they can go on an intensely violent spree, inflicting harm on themselves or others.

A strange behavior termed stereotypy is seen in those who

use amphetamines heavily. A simple act such as stringing beads, pacing the floor, cleaning, or shining shoes will be carried out repeatedly for hours. Amphetamines induce stereotypy in animals, too.

Experiencing the phenomenon called formication, the heavy amphetamine user hallucinates about the presence of insects crawling around just under the skin. So real is this hallucination that addicts have been known to probe with a knife in attempts to eliminate the crawling bugs. A skin mole may be watched for minutes to see if it will move. Formication also is seen in alcohol-induced delirium tremens and with heavy use of cocaine.

Desoxyn is indicated for use in children with attention-deficit disorder with hyperactivity. It is used in an overall program that also includes social, psychological, and educational elements. These children typically have short attention spans, emotional lability, impulsivity, and distractability. It is important that their diagnosis be carefully made and that the use of drugs really is necessary.

Drug testing for methamphetamine: In one study it was found that methamphetamine or amphetamine could be detected from 2 to 8 days in blood samples and from 17 to 36 days in urine samples following the last IV injection of methamphetamine. Although there obviously is considerable variation among abusers, these data should be helpful when testing employees or athletes for this drug. As discussed in the section on false positives, ephedrine, Ritalin, and antiobesity drugs and decongestants such as phenylpropanolamine and pseudoephedrine can give false positives in tests for amphetamines. To eliminate the possibility of such false positives, do not use these drugs for at least 1 month before you are scheduled to have the test done.

Abuse potential: high

Adverse effects: Methamphetamine raises blood pressure; it should be used with caution in people with even mild hypertension. If you are tired or feeling down, you should not use methamphetamine because the depression you will feel after the drug wears off will be worse than the original. Methamphetamine increases blood sugar, and diabetics who take it may discover that their diabetes is out of control. There is some evidence that children who are given amphetamines for many weeks or months do not achieve the gain in weight and height that they would have without the drug. This should be discussed with your physician. Tolerance to methamphetamine can easily occur when the drug is used for weeks or months to control obesity, and a psychological dependency is always a dangerous possibility. Methamphetamine should not be given to persons who have a history of drug abuse.

Drug interactions: The blood-lowering effects of guanethidine may be diminished by methamphetamine. Never combine a monoamine oxidase inhibitor such as Parnate or Nardil with any amphetamine, as dangerously high blood pressure may result. When a tricyclic antidepressant such as amitriptyline (Elavil) is combined with methamphetamine, overstimulation of the brain may occur. Phenothiazine tranquilizers such as Compazine, Temaril, or Thorazine can offset the brain-stimulant actions of amphetamines. Amphetamines can antagonize the hypotensive effects of methyldopa.

See also APPETITE-SUPPRESSANT DRUGS, AMPHETAMINES, DRUG TESTING, SYMPATHOMIMETICS

Methaqualone

Other names: Mandrax, Mequin, Parest, Quaalude, Sopor (all now removed from the market)
Source: synthesis
Pharmacology: nonbarbiturate sedative-hypnotic
Dose: 100-400 mg (when it was legal, methaqualone pills came in 150-, 200-, 300-, and 400-mg strengths)

When methaqualone, a nonbarbiturate sedative-hypnotic, was introduced in 1965, it was hailed as the long-awaited replacement for the dangerous barbiturates. Methaqualone was touted as a low-abuse-potential, addiction-free, safe, side-effect-free example of modern pharmacology. How tragically wrong that information was! Methaqualone ("ludes") has developed into one of our nation's greatest social hazards, involving medical and law-enforcement personnel from the local to the federal levels. Reaching its destructive zenith in 1980–81, when about 1 billion tablets a year were sold on the street, methaqualone earned its reputation as an "epidemic of horror." It threatens life from overdosage, serious or fatal accident, or a severe withdrawal syndrome that can include seizures. Methaqualone is no longer available from legitimate sources but still is sold illegally on the street.

Methaqualone (meth-ack'-kwa-lone) is chemically distinct from the barbiturates and has a greater variety of actions. It has antispasmodic, anticonvulsant, local anesthetic, and antitussive activity. Through its general depression of the CNS, it reduces heart rate, respiration, and muscular coordination. Five years after its introduction, however, it had become widely abused by American drug takers, who called it the "love drug." Methaqualone's explosive invasion of the drug culture stemmed in part from the popular view among abusers that it was a powerful aphrodisiac. But, as with alcohol, this effect is explained by the release of inhibitions as feelings of relaxation, confidence, and euphoria set in (abusers term this a high, but they are actually undergoing CNS depression).

Tolerance of and serious addiction to methaqualone can develop after a month's regular use. Regular use of 75 mg a day can easily swell to 750 mg a day; some abusers take 2000 mg a day. (Note that one cannot be sure what dose of a street drug one is ingesting. Street drugs don't come with guarantees of purity, strength, or effectiveness; in fact, some years ago there was an 82% rip-off rate on street methaqualone.) Abrupt withdrawal is characterized by severe *grand mal* seizures and is life-threatening. Hence detoxification is best carried out in a hospital. Since methaqualone and alcohol are metabolized by the same liver enzymes, the danger of overdosage from a combination of these two drugs is serious.

As methaqualone's bad reputation developed, licit manufacturers dropped it, one by one, until only the Lemmon Company remained; they changed the drug's trade name to Mequin. Ultimately, all legal manufacture was stopped, but existing stocks on shelves were allowed to remain. The supply vacuum was filled by illicit methaqualone tablets smuggled in from Colombia. Dealers in Colombia purchased bulk methaqualone from legitimate manufacturers in West Germany, Austria, Hungary, Switzerland, and the People's Republic of China. In the early 1980s, over 100 tons (1.2 billion 750-mg doses) of methaqualone entered the United States illegally each year. As federal narcotics agents cracked down, street prices soared to

$3.00–$5.00 per tablet, and in Las Vegas they sold for $7.00 apiece (their cost on legitimate prescription is 20 cents each). The largest areas of methaqualone abuse were in the Southeast and the Northeast. In Miami alone, two doctors grossed almost $700,000 in 13 months by setting up "stress clinics" and writing more than 6900 methaqualone prescriptions.

As Drug Abuse Warning Network (DAWN) data showed an alarming rate of methaqualone injuries, the DEA began diplomatic negotiations with the foreign countries that were supplying the bulk methaqualone to Colombia. This effort, plus meetings with international drug control agencies, reduced the flow of methaqualone to the United States but has hardly eliminated it. Methaqualone still ranks tenth on DAWN's list of hospital emergency room mentions.

In retrospect, we see a drug, introduced to an all-too-accepting medical profession as the safe answer to barbiturates, that turned out to be extremely addicting. This is another example of an approved drug that became a severe social hazard, readily found in schools, at parties, and in bars, that has cost our society hundreds of lives and billions of dollars.

Abuse potential: high

Adverse effects: Methaqualone is a sedative-hypnotic. That means it is a brain depressant, and when it is combined with alcohol there is a real danger of overdepression of the brain with consequent loss of coordination while walking, moving, or operating a car. But even uncombined use of methaqualone can be dangerous, for we know of coma produced by an overdose of 2.4 g and death following an 8-g dose. Development of tolerance to methaqualone with subsequent dependency is a threat as great as that with the barbiturates, and the withdrawal syndrome in a heavily addicted user can be life-threatening.

Drug interactions: Concurrent use of methaqualone with any brain depressant (alcohol, barbiturates, antihistamines, tranquilizers) can lead to oversedation in which physical coordination is lost; driving a car or operating machinery under this condition is extremely hazardous.

Methylphenidate. *See* RITALIN

Methyprylon. *See* NOLUDAR

Mickey Finn. *See* CHLORAL HYDRATE

Midol

Other names for ingredients: aspirin, cinnamedrine, caffeine
Source: compounding
Pharmacology: pain   reliever,   supposed   smooth-muscle
relaxant
Dose: Adult dose is 2 caplets, each containing 454 mg of
aspirin, 14.9 mg of cinnamedrine, and 32.4 mg of caffeine.

In some women menstruation is fraught with pain, cramping,
headache, irritability, tension, fluid accumulation, and back
pain. Midol is one of the heavily advertised products for the
treatment of these symptoms. Besides the original Midol formulation, which contains aspirin (for pain), cinnamedrine (smooth-
muscle relaxant), and caffeine (CNS stimulant, mild diuretic),
two new Midol products have appeared. In one, acetaminophen has replaced the aspirin, and in the other the only analgesic is ibuprofen. Ibuprofen is considered a better drug for dysmenorrhea than either aspirin or acetaminophen.

The FDA has ruled that the Midol product containing aspirin,
cinnamedrine, and caffeine lacks evidence of safety or effectiveness because of its cinnamedrine content (not effective at
this dose). Further, Pamabrom, found in the acetaminophen
formulation, is a minimally effective diuretic whose efficacy has
been questioned. In sum, the only effective ingredients in Midol
products are aspirin and acetaminophen. But why pay the high
Midol price for drugs you can buy cheaper generically? And if
you desire caffeine, drink coffee or tea.

Misuse potential: medium
Adverse effects: Aspirin can irritate the lining of the stomach
and cause nausea with minor blood loss into the intestine. Aspirin can interfere with blood clotting and should not be used
after surgery. A very small percentage of persons using aspirin

will be allergic to it, suffering pain, shock, or even death from a single dose. There is no way to predict who will suffer such an allergic reaction, although it is known that asthmatics are far more susceptible to an attack than nonasthmatics. Two caplets of Midol offer a heavy dose of aspirin; it is known that repeated large doses of aspirin can cause skin rashes, kidney damage, and changes in blood cells. If you take an acetaminophen-Midol product, the recommended dose of acetaminophen probably will not produce any significant adverse effects. Excessive doses, however, can lead to liver damage. The kidney also is sensitive to overdosage. CAUTION: Persons with a history of liver disease should avoid excessive use of acetaminophen and should restrict its use to 1 or 2 days.

The caffeine found in 2 Midol caplets is roughly equivalent to the amount you would receive if you drank 1½ cans of a cola beverage. In most people this will be of little consequence; in others, 64 mg of caffeine will cause agitation, restlessness, and possible insomnia.

Drug interactions: Aspirin interactions are common. Because of its very extensive use, aspirin has an increased chance of interacting with other drugs concurrently being taken. Aspirin combined with alcohol or with an anticoagulant can significantly increase bleeding tendency. Aspirin taken concurrently with oral antidiabetic drugs (such as Orinase or Diabinese) can result in too great a lowering of blood sugar. Aspirin will antagonize the systemic actions of the antiarthritic drugs Anturane and Benemid. If you are taking any prescription medication, consult your physician before heavily dosing yourself with aspirin.

Acetaminophen can increase the effects of concurrently administered oral anticoagulants. Combining alcohol with acetaminophen can increase the poisonous effects of both on the liver. Avoid these drug combinations, or consult your doctor beforehand.

See also MENSTRUAL PRODUCTS

Milk of Magnesia

Other names: magnesium hydroxide, 7.5% suspension in water; $Mg(OH)_2$

Source: compounding

Pharmacology: laxative, antacid

Dose: 15 ml (one-half fluid ounce, or 3 teaspoonfuls) as an antacid; 2–4 tablespoonfuls as a laxative; a 15-ml dose is equivalent to 3 tablets

We term milk of magnesia a laxative, but the more precise definition is saline cathartic. This means that after a dose most of it remains inside the intestine and attracts water to itself. The influx of water promotes peristalsis and more rapid evacuation of the bowel. Magnesium sulfate (Epsom salt) is another example of a saline cathartic.

Magnesium hydroxide is also well known for its antacid action. It is used in combination with aluminum hydroxide (Maalox, Mylanta, Gelusil), where its dual role is as antacid and laxative to counteract the constipating effects of the aluminum hydroxide.

Magnesium is an essential mineral in the human. It is found inside body cells as part of enzymes. A deficiency of magnesium can result in irritability of the nervous system, tremors, convulsions, and psychotic behavior, but an excess of magnesium can be dangerous, especially in persons with a history of kidney failure.

NOTE: The average healthy person who follows a sound diet will seldom if ever require either an antacid or a laxative. If one drinks plenty of water and consumes significant amounts of dietary fiber, the defecation process will take care of itself. The ads that urge us to make a laxative our "friend" or a "member of the family" are unconscionable. The more you depend on a laxative, the more dependent upon laxatives you will become.

CAUTION: Patients with kidney disorders should consult their physician before taking magnesium or aluminum preparations. Since magnesium hydroxide can bind drugs to its surface, always consult your physician before taking this antacid concurrently with any prescription drug. Drugs that bind to magnesium include indomethacin and digitalis.

Misuse potential: medium

Adverse effects: If one intends to use milk of magnesia as an antacid, and takes 2 or more of the 15-ml doses, one may experience unwanted laxative effects. Milk of magnesia puts a load on the kidneys, and people with kidney disorders should not use this product unless advised to by their physician. If you have abdominal pain, nausea, vomiting, or any other indication of appendicitis or obstructive disease, do not use this or any other laxative. CAUTION: Habitual use of laxatives—that is, for weeks at a time—can result in a dependence on them that is very difficult if not impossible to break. Very young children or newborns may not be able to handle magnesium products. A newborn died after being given a magnesium sulfate enema. If pregnant or nursing, consult a physician before using this product.

Drug interactions: Magnesium hydroxide is well known for its ability to bind drugs to its surface. That means that if you take it concurrently with a prescription drug, there is the possibility that the prescription drug will attach itself to the magnesium hydroxide, be excreted, and never do you any good. Drugs that bind to magnesium hydroxide include indomethacin (Indocin), chlorpromazine, and digitalis. Other drugs can bind, too—consult your physician before concurrent use of milk of magnesia and any prescription drug. Magnesium ion (along with calcium and aluminum) may diminish the absorption of tetracycline antibiotics. You can eliminate this interaction by spacing the doses 2–3 hours apart. Magnesium salts can potentiate the neuromuscular blocking actions of muscle relaxants such as succinylcholine, tubocurarine, and decamethonium. Vitamin D products may promote increased absorption of magnesium; in kidney failure patients this could cause problems of magnesium toxicity.

See also LAXATIVES

Mineral Oil

Other name: white petrolatum
Source: crude oil
Pharmacology: fecal softener
Dose: 1–3 tablespoonfuls
One of the fractions found in petroleum (crude oil) is mineral

oil, a colorless, clear liquid consisting of hydrocarbons from 18 to 24 carbons long. It has long been believed that mineral oil is chemically and physiologically inert, passing through the body unchanged, and that it is safe to use it as a laxative. In fact, it is widely used as an intestinal lubricant and stool softener. However, there is now enough evidence to conclude that mineral oil is not safe to use. The greatest hazard in its use is the danger of producing lipid pneumonia. This is a well-known condition in which some of the oil gets into the lungs either from oral ingestion or through use of oily nose drops and causes fluid accumulation in the lungs, with consequent impairment of breathing. Lying down (as at bedtime) after an oral dose of mineral oil can result in oil getting into the lungs. Mineral oil also is absorbed to a limited but significant extent from the intestines and gets into the lymph system, liver, and spleen. For more untoward actions, see the following discussion on adverse effects.

Mineral oil is another of the chemical crutches some people rely upon to support their neuroses, in this case the unrealistic anxiety about constipation. Consume a diet with a reasonable amount of fiber in it; drink plenty of water; and promptly respond to nature's call when it comes, and you will not require any laxative.

Misuse potential: medium

Adverse effects: Mineral oil, taken at mealtime or shortly thereafter, can dissolve vitamins A, D, E, and K from foods and carry them out of the body in the stool. Serious loss of vitamin A can cause night blindness and damage to the eye. Serious loss of vitamin D can reduce the body's ability to absorb and store calcium. The consequences of loss of vitamin E in man are not clear. Loss of vitamin K reduces the clotting ability of the blood. For the hemophiliac or patient taking an oral anticoagulant, this could have serious consequences. If you use mineral oil as a laxative, you may experience seepage of the oil from the anus with possibly an irritated anal sphincter. If you feel that you must use mineral oil, take only a small dose on an empty stomach, and do not lie down for at least a half hour after the dose. CAUTION: Do not use this or any other laxative if you have nausea, abdominal pain, or any sign of appendicitis.

Drug interactions: Laxatives speed up the movement of intestinal contents and can cause loss of medications taken by mouth. This is because there is less time for absorption from the gastrointestinal tract. Oral anticoagulants, vitamin K, and isoniazid are drugs that may fail to be absorbed if intestinal transit is speeded up.

See also LAXATIVES

MMDA. *See* HALLUCINOGENIC AMPHETAMINE DERIVATIVES

Morning Glory Seeds

Other name of active ingredient: lysergic acid amide
Source: plants
Pharmacology: hallucinogen
Dose of Seed: There is wide variation. From 4 to 40 seeds may be required to produce hallucinogenic effects, and these may be minimal.

These seeds do not contain LSD. They contain lysergic acid amide and other ergot alkaloids. (LSD is the N,N-diethylamide synthesized by Hofmann from lysergic acid; it doesn't exist as such in nature.)

Lysergic acid amide is the only psychoactive agent in morning glory seed. It has much less hallucinogenic and psychomotor activity than LSD and tends to produce sleepiness. There are many variations of morning glory plants; a large proportion are not hallucinogenic and contain no ergot alkaloids. In the early 1960s several varieties of California morning glory plants were discovered to be psychoactive. Named "heavenly blue" and "Pearly Gate," their seeds were purchased from seed and feed stores and consumed in large quantities. Federal agents seized many pounds of seeds in raids. Today one still occasionally hears of the use of morning glory, but mostly it is a drug of the past.

Ololiuqui—the seed of the morning glory *Rivea corymbusa*—was the ancient Aztec decoction employed by native priests to commune with their gods.

Abuse potential: medium
Adverse effects: There is a danger in taking very large doses of morning glory seeds. The ergot alkaloids contained therein

are powerful vasoconstrictors—that is, they clamp down on blood vessels, limiting blood flow. In some cases, the hands and feet are cold and numb, while in others, gangrene has developed from this lack of circulation. Operating a vehicle or machinery under the influence of this psychoactive drug can be hazardous.

Drug interactions: If a person has ingested a heavy dose of potent morning glory seeds and concurrently uses other brain stimulants such as epinephrine, amphetamines, or other hallucinogens, a dangerous psychotic state could be induced.

See also ERGOT, HALLUCINOGENS, PSYCHEDELICS

Morphine

Other name: morphine sulfate
Source: the plant *Papaver somniferum*
Pharmacology: narcotic analgesic (pain reliever)
Dose: 5–20 mg. Tablets are available containing 15 or 30 mg of morphine sulfate; suppositories contain 5, 10, or 20 mg. Injectables contain 2–10 mg/ml per milliliter.

The most important narcotic analgesic in opium is morphine, amounting to about 10% of opium's dry weight. Morphine, the first active ingredient ever to be isolated from a plant, was obtained as pure white crystals in 1803. Legally and pharmacologically morphine is a narcotic; it is classified as a Schedule II substance, which means it has medicinal value but high abuse potential.

Morphine's ability to relieve severe pain without causing loss of consciousness makes it an extremely useful drug. It can ease the pain of fractures, angina pectoris, surgery, kidney stone, gallstone, terminal illness, and trauma in general. The patient remains awake though often drowsy. Typical doses of morphine will not interfere with sensory perception (touching, hearing, vision) or speech (in contrast to alcohol). Morphine is especially effective in relieving dull pain, although in larger doses it also relieves sharp pain.

Morphine is an addicting drug, all the more so if it is taken by injection or in large doses. In one verified case an addict was taking 5000 mg of morphine daily, showing the remarkable tolerance that can be achieved with this opiate. Tolerance to one opiate—say, morphine—automatically confers tolerance to all other opiates (this is termed "cross-tolerance"). Three telltale signs diagnose a morphine addict (or any opiate addict): constriction of the pupil of the eye ("pinpoint pupil"), depression of respiration, and coma (if the addict has overdosed). Constipation is a common complaint in morphine addicts, the result of diminished bowel activity. Actually, this antiperistalsis effect is put to use in opiate treatment of diarrhea. Addicts also complain of diminished libido (sex drive). Because morphine depresses respiration, its use is contraindicated in bronchial asthma, acute alcoholism, any respiratory depression, oxygen lack, and cases of increased intracranial pressure.

Since addiction to morphine is a *physical* addiction, abruptly stopping use of the drug in an addict will lead to a physical withdrawal crisis. This is termed a withdrawal syndrome, can last for 6–10 days, and typically is characterized by a runny nose, nausea, vomiting, diarrhea, gooseflesh, uncontrollable yawning, severe sneezing, weakness, intestinal spasm, back pains, chills, uncontrolled orgasm, and severe tremors. Morphine withdrawal, however, usually is not life-threatening (as barbiturate or Valium withdrawal can be).

Abuse potential: high. Morphine does not give the intense euphoric "rush" observed with heroin but nonetheless is a very high abuse potential drug.

Adverse effects: If you are given morphine (or any opiate) for pain relief, you may experience nausea and/or vomiting. To overcome this, take the drug with food or ask your doctor if you can reduce the dose or take the drug less often. Serious overdosage with morphine is likely to cause the person to fall asleep or become stuporous, with a seriously depressed breathing rate and pupils pinpoint in size. Life can be threatened by morphine-induced respiratory depression, but the use of narcotic antagonists such as Narcan can restore adequate breathing. Long-term users of morphine, including addicts, report constipation and a diminished sex drive. If you are in a hospital and are given morphine for pain, your chances of becoming addicted are very small. The risk increases with increased size and frequency of dose, and especially if the drug is injected. As with any drug, the best advice is to take the smallest dose that will do the job, for the shortest time necessary.

Drug interactions: Combining morphine with other CNS depressants, including tranquilizers, can lead to oversedation. Patients receiving morphine and monoamine oxidase inhibitor drugs concurrently must be monitored for a possible crisis reaction.

See also METHADONE, NARCOTIC ANALGESICS, OPIATES, OPIUM, WITHDRAWAL

Mouthwash-Gargle Products

A visit to a large drugstore reveals the amazing variety of mouthwash-gargle products offered for sale. The following table lists four of the more popular along with their ingredients and comparative costs. Some of the products appear to be very highly priced, undoubtedly reflecting the cost of heavy advertising.

Ingredients in and cost of OTC Mouthwash-Gargle Products

Ingredient	Purpose	Brands and Their Ingredients*			
		Cēpacol	Listerine	Scope	Thrifty
cetylpyridinium chloride	antiseptic	yes	no	yes	no
denatured alcohol	solvent and antiseptic	yes 14%	yes 26.9%	yes 18.5%	yes 28.6%
saccharin	artificial sweetener	yes	no	yes	no
artificial colors	customer appeal	yes	caramel	yes	caramel
water	solvent	yes	yes	yes	yes
product cost per fluid ounce, approx.		15.0¢	12.5¢	16.6¢	6.2¢

*Other ingredients found in some products include flavoring agents, buffers, sobitol, detergents, polysorbates, domiphene bromide, glycerin, poloxamer 407, zinc chloride, and acetic acid.

Mouthwash-gargle preparations are advertised as treatments for odors of the mouth. Such odors can come from decaying food lodged between the teeth, or from infections of the upper respiratory tract. Using a mouthwash can eliminate an odor temporarily, but it makes more sense to get at the *cause* of the odor. Careful brushing of the teeth followed by cleansing with dental floss and rinsing with water will remove all food particles. Infections of the throat or nasopharyngeal region, if serious, require medical advice. Use of an OTC gargle in self-medication of a sore throat or upper respiratory tract infection is mostly a waste of time, since the gargle cannot contact enough of the infected area long enough to hasten the body's own natural healing process. Physicians recommend a salt-water gargle (compare costs) for certain upper respiratory infections.

Some mouthwash-gargle products are promoted as germ-killers ("kill bacteria by the millions on contact"). It's true that some preparations kill millions of microorganisms. What you are not told is that hundreds of millions of bacteria, yeasts, and viruses remain in the mouth and throat. Not only will the gargle not sterilize the oral cavity, it should not be expected to make you germ-free. Microorganisms in the mouth and throat are normal, as any mother of a teething baby knows. If you unfortunately have an infection of the gums (gingiva), trench mouth (Vincent's angina), or pyorrhea alveolaris, then you do, indeed, require an anti-infective, but one far more powerful than any OTC product can provide. Your physician can prescribe appropriate therapy for serious infections.

We discover a great similarity in the ingredients used in mouthwash-gargle products. Cetylpyridinium chloride NF, used in several of the preparations listed, is a surface-active agent with bactericidal properties. It is in the same category as benzalkonium chloride USP (Zephiran). Bactericidal effectiveness of agents such as cetylpyridinium chloride is diminished by dilution and by contact with body fluids and tissues. What is more, extended application time is needed to kill all bacteria. For example, a 0.1% solution of benzalkonium chloride applied to human skin requires about 7 minutes to kill half the bacteria present. Gargling or rinsing the mouth is a brief procedure that can eliminate only an insignificant number of microorganisms. The FDA has declared that cetylpyridinium chloride lacks evidence of both safety and effectiveness in use as a mouthwash/antiseptic.

It is an unfortunate comment on our society that mouthwash-gargle formulators see the necessity of including artificial colors and sweeteners in their products (and saccharin, at that).

In summary, mouthwash-gargle products offer little therapy. Their actions are temporary and generally do not correct the cause of the problem. If the ads convince you that you need a mouthwash, compare ingredients and consider using one of the cheaper brands that sell for half the cost of highly advertised brands.

Misuse *potential:* high

Adverse effects: Since mouthwash-gargle products are not supposed to be swallowed, there is little chance the chemicals they contain can harm you. The worst damage probably will be to your pocketbook.

MPTP

Other name: 1-Methyl-4-phenyl-1,2,5,6-tetrahydropyridine
Source: illicit synthesis
Pharmacology: street drug; can cause a disease similar to Parkinsonism
Dose: unknown

See the section on designer drugs. MPTP is a designer drug disaster. An underground chemist in some illicit California laboratory apparently attempted to synthesize MPPP, an analog (designer drug) of the well-known controlled opioid Demerol. Through an error in the synthesis the unexpected compound MPTP was produced, and when it hit the streets it produced a crippling condition that closely resembles Parkinsonism. Hundreds of drug abusers—mostly heroin addicts—who unknowingly ingested MPTP became violent, hallucinatory, and eventually brain-damaged and paralyzed. The condition appears to be irreversible. MPTP originally hit the streets as a tan or off-white powder but now is reported to be pure white and crystalline. It does not have the talcum consistency of fentanyl. Users have reported loss of memory, a burning sensation produced immediately after injection, drooling of saliva, sweating, and involuntary jerking of the arms and legs.

Scientists are very interested in this situation because they see possible clues to the explanation of the cause of Parkinsonism in the general population. Five legitimate chemists who worked with MPTP years before designer drugs were even dreamed of have come forward with the information that they have developed Parkinson symptoms to varying degrees. Here is an example of drug abusers unwittingly offering themselves as guinea pigs in drug testing, a protocol that is prohibited by law for the rest of the population.

In 1984 another Demerol analog (designer drug), 1-(2-phenylethyl)-4-phenylacetoxypiperidine (PEPAOP), was found in a sample of "synthetic" heroin. Its neurotoxicity is being studied.

Abuse potential: high

Adverse effects: This is a highly toxic drug and should be avoided at all costs. It irreversibly damages the brain, possibly producing a condition resembling that of Parkinsonism.

See also DESIGNER DRUGS

Mushrooms ('shrooms)

Other names: sacred mushrooms

Source: the fungus *Psilocybe mexicana* and other genera

Dose: Approximately 0.1 mg per kg of body weight. Not used in therapy. NOTE: There is no way of determining how much of the hallucinogen you are getting because there is absolutely no control of source, purity, or storage of these street drugs.

Psilocin and psilocybin are hallucinogenic alkaloids obtained from "sacred" mushrooms of Central America. The most important of the sacred mushrooms, long used by the mushroom-worshiping Indians of Mexico, is *Psilocybe mexicana* (other genera are *Conocybe* and *Stropharia*). Plant scientists believe that mushroom-eating and -worship was widespread, for stone images of mushrooms carved into the shape of a god date back to 1000 B.C. in Guatemala. Frescoes depicting the use of mushrooms have been found dating to A.D. 300. History's first recorded use occurred during the coronation feast of Montezuma in 1502.

Albert Hofmann, the discoverer of LSD, also investigated these Mexican mushrooms, determined the chemical structure of their active ingredients, and prepared the alkaloids synthetically. Psychotomimetics such as psilocin and psilocybin were often used in the 1950s and 1960s by writers, painters, and certain entertainers to achieve creativity, to release their "hidden potential," or just for thrills.

The hallucinatory experience produced by psilocybe alkaloids is roughly comparable to that produced by LSD, except that the LSD trip lasts about twice as long. Dangers involved stem not from physical harm but from the potential for inducing psychotic states that persist long after the expected end of the psychedelic experience. Tolerance to these hallucinogenic mushrooms (indeed, to most hallucinogens) quickly develops, and a period of about 5 days must elapse before the user can get high again.

On the street, the rip-off rate on supposedly hallucinogenic " 'shrooms" is strikingly high. Psilocybin (along with mescaline) heads the list of most often misrepresented hallucinogens, with less than 20% of the street samples actually containing psilocybin. Many of the mushrooms sold on the street are of the grocery store variety, frozen, and spiked with LSD or PCP.

Attempting to pick one's own mushrooms can be dangerous, since many species of mushrooms are highly poisonous.

Abuse potential: high

Adverse effects: Cases of *Psilocybe* mushroom poisoning have been reported in Washington and Oregon. Two adults and four children ate the mushrooms; all the children developed high fevers (102°–106°F), and one of the children died of convulsions. In spite of this, psilocybin is considered to be relatively nontoxic in man, at least at the doses that produce hallucinations. Of course, if one considers psychological effects, one could consider these agents to be highly toxic.

Drug interactions: Concurrent use of any brain stimulant such as epinephrine, amphetamines, or hallucinogenic amphetamine derivatives could induce a dangerous psychotic state.

See also HALLUCINOGENS, PSYCHEDELICS

Mylanta. *See* ANTACIDS

N

Nandrolone. *See* ANABOLIC STEROIDS, STEROIDS

Narcotic Analgesics

Other names: opiate or opioid painkiller
Source: plants or syntheses
Pharmacology: painkillers, cough suppressants, antidiarrheals
Dose: variable

One can consider "narcotic analgesics" from both a legal and a pharmacological viewpoint. Pharmacologically, a narcotic analgesic is an opiate or opioid that acts on the CNS to relieve pain without necessarily producing unconsciousness; it also causes drowsiness, changes in mood, mental clouding, apathy, and lethargy. One of the most common adverse effects of narcotic analgesics is nausea and vomiting; all of these drugs cause this to some extent, and it limits their usefulness.

The federal Comprehensive Drug Abuse Prevention and Control Act of 1970 (and the many state laws patterned after it) defines narcotic drugs as opium, opiates, and their salts, derivatives, or preparations, whether produced directly or indirectly by extraction from substances of vegetable origin, or independently by means of chemical synthesis, or by a combination of both. Coca leaves and cocaine also are included in the 1970 Act as narcotic drugs! Pharmacologically this makes no sense, for cocaine is a powerful CNS stimulant, not a depressant like the opiates. Nonetheless, legally cocaine is a narcotic drug, and courts have held that it is valid to classify cocaine as a narcotic for purposes of prosecution.

The table on pages 184–86 lists narcotic analgesic drugs and preparations available by prescription or OTC. Note that heroin is not included because it is not legally available in any form in this country. Many of these drugs are also discussed in their own sections. Note that all have medium to high abuse potential—that is, may be habit-forming.

All narcotic analgesics are classified as Schedule II controlled substances under the 1970 Controlled Substances Act. Possession, distribution, transportation, sale, or offering for sale without a prescription or other authorization are punishable by jail sentence and/or fines. Terpin Hydrate and Codeine Elixir and paregoric are "exempt narcotics" because of their low opiate content.

Abuse potential: high

Adverse effects: All opium-related compounds, whether naturally occurring or synthetic, can depress respiration to some degree. This becomes an important factor only when overdosage has occurred, but not in normal, prescribed doses. These drugs also cause nausea and vomiting, especially when the user is up and about. See the individual sections for further discussion.

Drug interactions: Avoid combining these drugs with other central nervous system depressants such as sleeping pills and tranquilizers, as oversedation could occur. Do not take a monoamine oxidase inhibitor such as Parnate or Nardil in combination with any of these drugs, as a possible crisis reaction may occur. NOTE: Do not substitute one narcotic painkiller for another without the approval of your physician, as some combinations work against each other.

See also the individual sections

Nasal Decongestants. *See* COLD REMEDIES

Nembutal. *See* BARBITURATES

Generic Name	Other Name	Comments
alphaprodine	Nisentil	Injectable; given intravenously, 0.5 mg/kg.
butorphanol	Stadol	Injectable. Dose: 2 mg.
codeine	—	Usually comes in combination with acetaminophen or aspirin; dose for pain relief: 30–120 mg; for cough suppression: 10–30 mg. Discussed in its own section.
concentrated opium alkaloids	Pantopon	Injectable; morphine makes up half of total alkaloid content. Dose: 5–20 mg.
dihydrocodeine bitartrate	Compal, Synalgos-DC	Semisynthetic; related to codeine. May be dispensed in combination with either aspirin or acetaminophen.
Terpin Hydrate and Codeine Elixir	T.H. & C.E.	In some states sold OTC. For cough suppression. Dose: 1 teaspoonful. Not for children under 12 years.
fentanyl	Sublimaze	Very widely used in surgery. Discussed in its own section.
hydrocodone	Hycodan, Vicodin	Hycodan used as a cough suppressant, Vicodin for pain relief. Dose: 5 mg (1 tablet).
hydromorphone	Dilaudid	Use in pregnancy only with doctor's permission. Five times as potent as morphine; oral dose: 2 mg.

Generic Name	Other Name	Comments
levorphanol	Levo-Dromoran	Average adult dose: 2 mg (1 tablet).
meperidine	Demerol	Typical dose: 80–100 mg; lasts 2–4 hours. Discussed in its own section.
methadone	Dolophine	Key drug in heroin detoxification and methadone maintenance. Discussed in its own section.
morphine	M.S.	Dose: 5–20 mg. Most abundant of the opium alkaloids. Discussed in its own section.
nalbuphine	Nubain	Injectable for relief of moderate to severe pain. Dose: 10 mg.
oxycodone	Percodan, Percocet	Aspirin-allergic persons should know that Percodan also contains a standard dose of aspirin. Percocet contains acetaminophen rather than aspirin. Dose: 4.5 mg (1 tablet).
oxymorphone	Numorphan	Injectable. Semisynthetic substitute for morphine. Dose: 1 mg by injection.
paregoric	camphorated tincture of opium	In some states sold OTC. For relief of diarrhea. Discussed in its own section.

Generic Name	Other Name	Comments
pentazocine	Talwin	Often used as a preoperative medication. Dose: 30 mg by injection. Discussed in its own section.
propoxyphene	Darvon	Available in combination with aspirin and acetaminophen. Sold generically. Usual dose: 65 mg. Discussed in its own section.

Neosporin

Other names of active ingredients: polymyxin B, bacitracin, neomycin

Source: microorganisms

Pharmacology: anti-infective

Dose: applied locally 2–5 times a day

Neosporin is the proprietary name for a mixture of three antibiotics: polymyxin B, bacitracin, and neomycin. Neosporin ointment is sold on prescription and OTC as a first aid to help prevent bacterial infection in minor cuts, burns, and abrasions. Neosporin Ophthalmic Ointment is a prescription-only item intended for short-term use in superficial, external eye infections.

Theoretically, combining three antibiotics, each with its own spectrum of antibacterial activity, should provide superior bactericidal coverage. In practice, many variables can affect the therapeutic outcome, including how much of the medication is applied, how often, accidental loss, bacterial resistance, and the development of allergic response. Very likely, thorough washing of the injured area immediately after the trauma will be just as effective as the ointment.

The wisdom of using antibiotics without medical supervision has been long questioned. Neomycin has clear potential for toxicity to the ear and kidney. Bacterial resistance can develop when insufficient antibiotic is used. Deep or puncture wounds are difficult or impossible to treat with a topical product, and the user may be lulled into a false sense of security that the ointment is providing protection.

Misuse potential: medium

Adverse effects: Neomycin, one ingredient in the OTC ointment, has a history of causing skin allergies; if your skin becomes red after use or fails to heal, you might be sensitive and should stop using this product. If this product gets into the bloodstream (by absorption through broken skin), it can cause damage to the kidneys. For this reason do not use Neosporin ointment on large skin surfaces unless directed by your physician. Do not use this product in the ear if the eardrum is perforated. CAUTION: Neosporin ointment is not the same as Neosporin ophthalmic ointment, sterile; only the latter should be used in the eyes.

Drug interactions: Do not use neomycin concurrently with other antibiotics (such as streptomycin or dihydrostreptomycin) that can also damage the nerves that control hearing, since the effects might be additive.

See also ANTIBIOTICS

Nicorette

Other name of active ingredient: nicotine
Source: prescription only
Pharmacology: antismoking chewing gum
Dose: 1 stick of gum (contains 2 mg of nicotine)

The FDA has approved the first antismoking chewing gum, Nicorette, as an aid in eliminating nicotine dependency. Available only by prescription, the gum is chewed when the smoker feels the urge for a cigarette. Each stick of gum contains 2 mg of nicotine bound to an ion-exchange resin. Chewing hastens release of the nicotine; "parking" the gum in the buccal cavity slows release.

Does the gum work to control smoking? Apparently yes, say researchers who have studied its use in Europe and Canada. In one double-blind study, 28% of users were able to stay off cigarettes for up to 1 year. The gum is most advantageously used by highly motivated people who also participate in some form of behavior modification program. Ninety-six sticks of gum cost about $20.

Misuse potential: low

Adverse effects: If this gum is used by a smoker who is already heavily dosed with nicotine, there will be no additional threats to health. If this gum is chewed by a person who is free of nicotine, the following reactions can possibly be expected: nausea, vomiting, headache, rapid heartbeat, rise in blood pressure, and sweating. The faster you chew the gum the faster the nicotine is released and the more likely you are to experience its adverse effects.

CAUTION: Keep this gum away from children; not to be used by pregnant women or ex-smokers who wish to remain free of nicotine addiction. Nicotine products are contraindicated in persons with a history of heart or cardiovascular disease, peptic ulcer, or irritations of the mouth. NOTE: Not more than 30 sticks of 2-mg gum should be chewed in any 24-hour period.

Drug interactions: Nicotine ingestion, whether by smoking or gum, can stimulate the liver to produce enzymes that can cross over and speed up the breakdown of other drugs, including caffeine, theophylline, imipramine (Tofranil), and pentazocine (Talwin). Conversely, if one abruptly stops nicotine intake, the blood levels of all of these drugs—and some others as well— can unexpectedly rise. Concurrent use of nicotine and the diuretic furosemide can result in reduced action of the latter. Likewise, combining nicotine and propranolol (Inderal) can result in decreased heart output and increased blood pressure. Nicotine can increase circulating levels of cortisol and the catecholamines (epinephrine, norepinephrine, and dopamine).

See also NICOTINE

Nicotine

Other name: none

Source: the plant *Nicotiana tabacum*

Pharmacology: CNS, respiratory, and heart stimulant; nauseant; peripheral vasoconstrictor

Dose: not used medicinally: Nicorette chewing gum contains 2 mg per stick. A 1-pack-a-day smoker is exposed to about 18 mg of nicotine.

Nicotine, the most abundant of the 12 volatile alkaloids in

tobacco leaf, is partly destroyed at the temperature of a burning cigarette, but on the average about 0.9 mg of it per cigarette still is delivered to the smoker's lungs.

Nicotine is one of the most poisonous of all drugs we routinely take into our bodies. A 60-mg dose has been known to cause death in humans; it acts about as fast as cyanide. Pharmacologically, nicotine excites the CNS at all levels and can produce tremors in the extremities. It also markedly increases respiration and heart rate, increases blood pressure, constricts peripheral blood vessels (leading to cold hands and feet), stimulates the release of epinephrine, causes nausea and vomiting, and elevates concentrations of free fatty acids (implicated in hardening of the arteries). The heart and vascular system bear the brunt of the strong effects of nicotine, probably explaining the clearcut association between cigarette smoking and cardiovascular disease. Cigarette smokers inhale nicotine and also the tars and cancer-causing agents present in the cigarette smoke. They may experience irritation of the throat and bronchi, diminished vital capacity because of lung deterioration, and—if they are pregnant women—damage to the fetus that results in impaired growth and a low birth weight.

Many authorities now consider nicotine a powerfully addicting drug, capable of inducing tolerance and even a mild withdrawal syndrome in heavy users. The majority of heavy smokers are compulsive about their smoking, preoccupied with obtaining a supply of their drug, experience extreme difficulty in stopping smoking, and exhibit a strong tendency to relapse after having quit. The would-be tobacco abstainer now can obtain nicotine in the form of a prescription chewing gum (Nicorette), each stick of which contains 2 mg of nicotine bound to an ion-exchange resin (see the section on Nicorette). Chewing hastens release of the nicotine, while "parking" the gum in the buccal cavity (between the teeth and cheek) slows release. Nicotine skin patches have been developed, and they work, but they are not on the market yet.

Concentrated extracts of tobacco have long been used in horticulture as insecticides and fungicides, especially in plant sprays. The extracts contain high concentrations of nicotine. Unfortunately, such sprays are sometimes stored in old beverage containers in the family garage, where young children mistake them for a pleasant drink, with tragic results.

One must distinguish between the alkaloid nicotine and the antipellagra vitamin nicotinic acid. The latter can be obtained by chemical oxidation of the former, but they are not the same substance in any sense.

Abuse potential: high

Adverse effects: Nicotine comes in the form of cigarette smoke (which is typically inhaled deep into the lungs), pipe smoke (which affects mostly the oral cavity), smokeless or chewing tobacco (which affects the mouth), and chewing gum (which affects the mouth). Thus the adverse effects that one may experience can differ depending upon the form and whether smoke is a factor. The nicotine that enters the bloodstream, however, can produce predictable effects. Nicotine stimulates the release of epinephrine with consequent increase in heart rate and blood pressure. The brain and spinal cord are stimulated, with possible induction of fine tremors in the hands, increased respiration rate, nausea, and vomiting. Circulation in the fingers and toes is cut down, but the gastrointestinal tract can be stimulated with the possible production of diarrhea.

Drug interactions: Nicotine can have a strong effect on the action of prescription drugs that the smoker is taking concurrently. For example, Darvon can lose its pain-killing effect in a smoker, and tranquilizers such as Valium may work with diminished frequency. Smokers have been known to require 1½ to 2 times as much theophylline, an important bronchodilator used in treating asthma, as nonsmokers to achieve the same effects. The half-life of theophylline is reduced to about 4 hours (from about 7 hours in the nonsmoker). How are these effects explained? Some researchers believe that nicotine stimulates the liver to increase its production of enzymes responsible for the metabolism of many drugs and chemicals, including pain relievers, tranquilizers, and theophylline. As a consequence, the rate of drug metabolism is accelerated, with decreased intensity and duration of action. Regardless of theories, we are sure of this: With certain drugs, smokers need different doses or different frequency of administration than nonsmokers, and when smokers stop their consumption, their drug regimen may need adjustment. Note the following list of interactions between smoking and drugs presumably based on alterations in drug metabolism.

Analgesics
- propoxyphene (Darvon): higher rates of ineffective responses
- antipyrene: increased hepatic metabolism
- phenacetin: lower plasma levels
- pentazocine: higher maintenance dose needed

Tricyclic antidepressants
- imipramine (Tofranil): increased clearance rate

Xanthines
- theophylline: significantly accelerated metabolism

Tranquilizers
- diazepam (Valium): CNS depression less frequent (probably due to increased rate of metabolism)
- chlorpromazine (Thorazine): reduced drowsiness

Oral contraceptive users who smoke have a far greater risk of cardiovascular morbidity than nonsmokers, and this risk is worsened by age. For example, the risk of fatal heart attack in women Pill users in the 30–39-year age group is 10 times greater in smokers than in nonsmokers.

By law, smokeless tobacco (chewing tobacco) packages must now carry a warning of the danger of cancer of the mouth. Such carcinogenicity probably is not due to nicotine alone, but to other tobacco leaf constituents either in combination with nicotine or alone.

See also ADDICTION, ORAL CONTRACEPTIVES, WITHDRAWAL

Nitrates. *See* NITRITES

Nitrites

Other names: amyl nitrite, butyl nitrite, Isoamyl nitrite, pearls, poppers
Source: chemical preparation
Pharmacology: vasodilator, antidote in cyanide poisoning
Dose: 0.3 ml (approximately 6 drops) by inhalation

Nitrites (as exemplified by amyl nitrite, $C_5H_{11}NO_2$) and nitrates (as exemplified by nitroglycerin) have similar actions in the body. Both are vasodilators—that is, they increase the size or inner diameter of blood vessels, especially arteries and capillaries, allowing a greater flow of oxygen-rich blood to body tissues. Simultaneously, they cause a drop in blood pressure, due, of course, to the increased volume of the cardiovascular system.

Vasodilators such as amyl nitrite, nitroglycerin, erythrityl tetranitrate (Cardilate), isosorbide dinitrate, and pentaerythritol tetranitrate (Peritrate) are especially useful in treating the pain of angina pectoris, a condition in which the blood vessels supplying oxygen to heart muscle have become narrowed with age or disease. Dilation of these arteries allows more blood to the heart and temporarily relieves the pain.

Amyl nitrite has become a drug of abuse, used to enhance sexual response and pleasure. Its vasodilator action presumably prolongs the pleasure of orgasm in males. In others it is inhaled to produce a giddy "high," which in reality is the dizziness associated with a dramatic fall in blood pressure. A throbbing headache may result from expanded blood vessels in the brain. Amyl nitrite is sold in cloth-covered glass vials ("poppers," "snappers"), which are broken in the hand and the volatile liquid contents inhaled.

Two other nitrites, butyl nitrite and isobutyl nitrite, are also sold in porno and head shops and elicit the same pharmacological response as amyl nitrite. They are sold as "Locker Room" and "Rush."

Amyl nitrite is a volatile, yellowish liquid with an etherlike odor and a pungent taste. It is very flammable and forms explosive mixtures with air. It does not last long in the body, since the liver rapidly metabolizes it.

Amyl nitrite is used to treat cyanide poisoning; it is administered first by inhalation, followed by the intravenous route.

Nitrites and nitrates are not acutely poisonous in the human. However, their long-term use as preservatives in meats (sodium nitrate) has been criticized as a possible cause of cancer of the GI tract.

Abuse potential: high

Adverse effects: When amyl nitrite is inhaled, it rapidly enters the bloodstream and is distributed to all parts of the body, where it dilates blood vessels and causes a significant drop in blood pressure. The user can become dizzy to the point of falling down. A severe headache may also be experienced. Postural hypotension may be seen, in which suddenly standing up may cause a big drop in blood pressure and extreme dizziness. Amyl nitrite has been known to cause visual problems—for example, the user may see halos of yellow or blue that surround a dark object when viewed against a light background.

Drug interactions: If you are already taking a drug for high blood pressure and you combine it with any nitrite, you may experience a dangerous fall in blood pressure leading to unconsciousness. Because alcohol also is a vasodilator, concurrent use of it with any nitrite can produce a dangerous fall in blood pressure.

Nitrous Oxide

Other names: laughing gas, N_2O
Source: chemical decomposition of ammonium nitrate
Pharmacology: inhalation anesthetic
Dose: variable

Nitrous oxide has been used in inhalation anesthesia for 100 years and continues to have wide application in hospitals and in the practice of dental surgery. In hospital operations, N_2O is typically administered by inhalation with oxygen and other anesthetics; it is not a potent agent, and its effects wear off rather quickly. It is nonflammable, a nonirritant, and pleasant-smelling.

Nitrous oxide is a common drug of abuse. This gas is inhaled from cylinders, balloons that have been filled with it, or from aerosol cans in which it is used as a propellant. Nitrous oxide induces pleasurable sensations, including auditory illusions, giddiness, exhilaration, or disinhibition. Users say they can get "high" on it. Although nitrous oxide obviously is not acutely poisonous, there always is the possibility that the abuser will inhale so much of it (to the exclusion of oxygen) that irreversible brain damage will result. If N_2O is inhaled while driving a car or engaging in some physical activity, there is the possibility of physical injury.

Abuse potential: medium
Adverse effects: There are literature reports that link nitrous

oxide with infertility, birth defects, and spontaneous abortion. These, however, are from chronic exposure, as in the workplace. The occasional, minor inhalation of nitrous oxide probably will produce no significant bad effects.

CAUTION: Persons who have asthma, emphysema, pulmonary disease, or other conditions that deprive them of oxygen are at high risk if they inhale any gas or volatile substance. In doses large enough to produce anesthesia, nitrous oxide will depress respiration.

Drug interactions: Respiratory depressants such as morphine will act additively to nitrous oxide.

Noludar

Other name: methyprylon
Source: synthesis
Pharmacology: hypnotic (sleep aid)
Dose: individualized. Usually for adults 1 capsule of 300 mg strength or 1–2 tablets of 200 mg strength before retiring. Use in children is highly individualized.

Chemically, Noludar is neither a barbiturate nor a benzodiazepine-type minor tranquilizer, although it is similar in its action to the barbiturates. Noludar is a "downer" that is widely used as a sleep aid. It is a cyclic imide that closely resembles the now-outlawed methaqualone (Quaalude); it induces sleep in 40 minutes in patients with simple insomnia, and the sleep lasts 5–8 hours.

The danger with Noludar, as with so many sleep-inducing agents, lies in the great temptation to use, reuse, and finally overrely. It is just too easy to get to depend upon a chemical for sleep. And with Noludar, there is a real risk of developing a dependency, either physical or psychological, with a significant withdrawal syndrome when the drug is finally discontinued. People who have a history of alcohol or drug dependence should probably not be given Noludar. In any event, do not use this drug for more than 7 days; preferably use it only once or twice occasionally if you must.

Abuse potential: medium
Adverse effects: Do not take more than 400 mg of Noludar in any one day; use caution in operating a car or machinery while

under the influence of this drug. Safety of use in children under 12 years has not been established. There have been reports of hallucinations produced by this drug. Methyprylon is a Schedule III drug—it can induce tolerance and physical dependence in the heavy user, similar to that produced by the barbiturates. Hence prolonged or heavy use should be strictly avoided. Use this drug with caution if you have kidney or liver disease. Pregnancy category B. Pregnant women should use this drug only with the approval of their physician, as should nursing mothers.

Numerous types of adverse reactions are possible with this drug. They include mental confusion, depression, anxiety, nightmares, blurred vision, nausea, diarrhea, constipation, rash, and generalized allergic reaction. See your physician if these reactions develop.

Drug interactions: The concomitant use of alcohol and Noludar can produce dangerous brain depression; this combination must be avoided. The effects of methyprylon are additive to those of other brain depressants and the narcotic analgesics such as Demerol. Noludar stimulates the liver to produce enzymes that can cross over and speed up the breakdown of other prescription drugs, including barbiturates.

See also SLEEP AIDS

Nose Drops. *See* COLD REMEDIES

Novahistine DMX Cough and Cold Formula Decongestant

Novahistine DMX Decongestant

Other names of active ingredients: dextromethorphan, pseudoephedrine

Source: compounding

Pharmacology: cough suppressant, nasal decongestant

Dose: 2 teaspoonfuls every 4 to 6 hours for adults and children 12 years and older; 1 teaspoonful every 4 to 6 hours for children 6–12 years; ½ teaspoonful every 4 to 6 hours for children 2–6 years of age. Limit doses to not more than 4 in any 24-hour period. Do not give to children under 2 years of age without the approval of a physician.

In addition to dextromethorphan and pseudoephedrine, this product contains 10% alcohol (that's 20 proof), and the supposed expectorant guaifenesin. However, the FDA has determined that guaifenesin lacks evidence of safety and effectiveness as an expectorant.

Novahistine DMX is another example of a "shotgun" preparation that, like pellets from a shotgun, is likely to hit something at the expense of much wasted therapeutic effort. No ingredient in this product will cure a cold or even speed up your recovery. For the consumer, the problem with shotgun formulas is that you must expose yourself to many drugs to get the possible benefits of one. For example, if you wish to treat a cough with the dextromethorphan in this product, you must also ingest a potent central nervous system stimulant (pseudoephedrine) and 20-proof alcohol, not to mention the probably useless guaifenesin. (See the following discussion for possible adverse effects).

Note that a productive cough should not necessarily be treated with a cough suppressant. A productive cough is the body's means of eliminating potentially troublesome fluid accumulation. Novahistine DMX is indicated for dry coughs. However, a persistent dry cough may be a sign of trouble; consult your physician.

Misuse potential: medium

Adverse effects: The pseudoephedrine contained in this product is the ingredient most likely to cause problems. It is intended to act as a vasoconstrictor that will produce temporary relief of nasal congestion, but it also can stimulate the heart, vascular system, and brain. While in most people its adverse effects are minor to nonexistent, in susceptible people it deserves serious consideration. Elderly persons (over 60 years) may be especially sensitive to pseudoephedrine, as can be the very young. Nursing mothers can pass the drug along to their baby in breast milk. You should avoid any pseudoephedrine-containing product if you are pregnant, have high blood pressure, diabetes mellitus, heart disease, glaucoma, hyperthyroidism, or an enlarged prostate. If you have serious hardening of the arteries or severe coronary artery disease, do not use this product. Users of this product occasionally report upset stomach, nausea, a too-fast heart rate, palpitations, dizziness, restlessness, headache, insomnia, anxiety, hallucinations, and convulsions.

Drug interactions: If pseudoephedrine is combined with a monoamine oxidase inhibitor such as Parnate or Nardil, a serious hypertensive crisis can occur. Avoid this combination of drugs. The pseudoephedrine in this product can counteract the effects of antihypertensive drugs such as methyldopa, mecamylamine, reserpine, and the veratrum alkaloids. Taken concurrently with other sympathomimetics (such as epinephrine), pseudoephedrine can cause excessive stimulation of the cardiovascular system.

See also PSEUDOEPHEDRINE.

Nupercainal Ointment, Suppositories

Other name of active ingredient: dibucaine
Source: synthesis
Pharmacology: local anesthetic
Dose: suppository: 1 after each bowel movement, not to exceed 6 in 24 hours

The ointment, promoted for pain relief, contains the local anesthetic dibucaine. The suppository, sold for the temporary relief of itching and discomfort of hemorrhoids, contains the local anesthetic dibucaine, zinc oxide, cocoa butter, and bismuth subgallate. NOTE: The FDA has concluded that the suppository form lacks evidence of safety and effectiveness in at least 1 ingredient, the combination of ingredients, or the dosage form.

In spite of all of the advertising hoopla, these suppositories are of little proven value in the treatment of hemorrhoids. Dibucaine is an effective local anesthetic, but not a lot of it is going to act on the actual hemorrhoidal tissue when the suppository is inserted into the anus. Most will slip on by before it melts with the body heat. Also, a local anesthetic can give little more than some temporary relief; it cannot heal the condition. And the makers themselves state that these suppositories are not for prolonged use.

Misuse potential: high

Adverse effects: CAUTION: Poisoning can occur if Nupercainal suppositories are swallowed, especially by children. It is important that you avoid contact of this product with the eyes. This product is not for prolonged use.

See also HEMORRHOIDAL PRODUCTS

Nutmeg

Other name of active ingredient: myristicin
Source: plant
Pharmacology: hallucinogen
Dose: 6–8 tablespoonfuls

Known as a condiment to millions of people around the world, nutmeg (from the seeds of the tree *Myristica fragrans*) produces mild hallucinogenic effects in some people. This effect was unknown until the 1960s, but since then it has been experienced by students and prisoners. In some prisons, nutmeg has had to be removed from the kitchens because of widespread abuse. The nutmeg discussed here is the same as that sold in any grocery store.

The hallucinogenic effect of nutmeg is unpredictable owing to variations in potency in batches or to differences in users, but it is capable of producing qualitatively a response similar to that of LSD or mescaline. Its onset of action is from 2 to 5 hours, a delay the naïve user does not anticipate.

Nutmeg contains myristicin and elemicin, chemicals related to eugenol and somewhat more distantly to mescaline.

Abuse potential: medium

Adverse effects: The large dose of nutmeg required to produce the psychotropic response probably will induce nausea and vomiting, but if the user can retain the drug in his or her body, there probably will be dizziness, dry mouth, headache, and a rapid heartbeat.

Drug interactions: Concurrent use of any brain stimulant such as epinephrine, dopamine, an amphetamine or any hallucinogenic amphetamine derivative can induce a dangerous psychotic state.

See also HALLUCINOGENS

NyQuil Nighttime Colds Medicine

Other names of active ingredient: acetaminophen, doxylamine, pseudoephedrine, dextromethorphan

Source: compounding

Pharmacology: pain and fever reliever, antihistamine, nasal decongestant, cough suppressant

Dose: For adults and children 12 years and over, 2 table-spoonfuls at bedtime. This product is not recommended for children.

From the name "Colds Medicine" one might get the idea that NyQuil will cure a head cold. However, there is no cure for the common head cold. Nonetheless, the very heavily advertised NyQuil continues to appeal to millions of Americans who believe it is doing them some good.

NyQuil is but one of the many "shotgun" cold products on the market. It contains drugs having 4 distinct pharmacological actions, plus 25% (50-proof) alcohol. NyQuil contains acetaminophen (pain and fever reliever), doxylamine (like all antihistamines, considered to be ineffective in preventing or aborting the common cold), pseudoephedrine (nasal decongestant), and dextromethorphan (cough suppressant). This shotgun approach would be appropriate if one had pain, fever, allergy, stuffed-up nose, and a cough all at once! NyQuil is an expensive, contrived product that most cold sufferers do not need and do not fully make use of. It makes more sense to treat individual symptoms with individual drugs, or with nondrug approaches, as the occasion arises. What is more, if one takes a multidrug product like NyQuil, one is exposed to a possible multitude of adverse effects or allergic responses.

Because it contains so many ingredients, NyQuil is not to be taken if you plan to operate a car or machinery, if you have high blood pressure, heart or thyroid disease, or diabetes mellitus. If you are a recovering alcoholic, the last product you would want to take is 50-proof NyQuil.

The pseudoephedrine in this product is a potent sympathomimetic. It can cause dizziness and nervousness. This product should not be used by children under 12 years of age. Each fluid ounce of NyQuil contains 1000 mg of acetaminophen, a very heavy dose. See the section on acetaminophen for its potential for causing liver damage.

NyQuil is widely used by insomniacs who go through bottle after bottle of it, week after week. It induces sleep because three of its ingredients—doxylamine, dextromethorphan, and alcohol—are all CNS depressants. It is all too easy to become habituated to and then dependent upon such a chemical combination to get to sleep each night. Users should be aware of this fact.

NyQuil is very expensive. Its ingredients can be purchased singly and generically at half the price or less.

Abuse potential: high

Adverse effects: If you do not exceed the recommended doses for acetaminophen, you probably will not experience any significant adverse effects. However, excessive doses, especially of the extra-strength preparations, can lead to liver damage. The kidney also is sensitive to overdosage. CAUTION: Persons with a known history of liver disease should avoid excessive use of acetaminophen and should restrict its use to brief periods.

Some people who take doxylamine will experience dryness of the mouth, dizziness, difficulty in urination, nausea, vomiting, and double vision.

Pseudoephedrine should be used cautiously in people who have hypertension, heart disease, diabetes, or a hypersensitivity to ephedrine. Pseudoephedrine can cause restlessness, insomnia, and dryness of the mouth and throat. Long-term use of any nasal shrinker is to be avoided.

Drug interactions: Combining alcohol with acetaminophen can increase the poisonous effects of both on the liver. Either avoid these drug combinations, or consult your doctor beforehand.

Concurrent use of alcohol with any antihistamine can result in dangerous sedation of the brain.

Simultaneous use of pseudoephedrine and monoamine oxidase inhibitor drugs can result in serious intensified action of pseudoephedrine. Pseudoephedrine can reduce the antihypertensive effects of methyldopa and reserpine.

See also ACETAMINOPHEN, ANTIHISTAMINES, PSEUDOEPHEDRINE, DEXTROMETHORPHAN

O

Opiates

Narcotic analgesics that have their origin in opium are termed opiates. Examples are morphine, codeine, heroin (made by acetylation of morphine), oxycodone (Percodan), hydromorphine (Dilaudid), and Pantopon. Opium consists of the dried sap collected from the unripe seed capsule of the opium poppy.

Synthetic narcotic analgesics such as meperidine (Demerol), methadone (Dolophine), pentazocine (Talwin), fentanyl (Sublimaze), and bupremorphine (Buprenex) are termed opioids. Whether natural or synthetic, all these narcotics act at the same place in the brain and are listed in Schedule II of the 1970 Controlled Substances Act (see the section on controlled substances). They comprise the so-called hard narcotics.

All opiates and opioids have the potential for inducing tolerance and physical dependence in the user. Heroin, with its pleasureful "rush" upon injection, is highly addictive. There is crossover tolerance among all members of the group. A serious withdrawal crisis occurs when an addict is abruptly denied any of these drugs.

Manufacture, possession, or distribution of any of these drugs without a legal prescription or other authorization subjects one to possible first-time imprisonment of up to 15 years and/or a $25,000 fine. Second-offense convictions carry twice the penalties. The 1970 Act provides for a possible 1-year probation for a first-time offender caught in simple possession. Also for a first-time offender under 21 years, the record of arrest may be expunged, restoring the person to the legal status he or she had before conviction.

See also CODEINE, MORPHINE, NARCOTIC ANALGESICS, OPIUM, WITHDRAWAL

Opium

Other names of active ingredients: morphine, codeine
Source: the opium poppy plant
Pharmacology: narcotic analgesic, cough suppressant
Dose: opium as such is used only in paregoric (see that section)

The opium poppy plant, *Papaver somniferum,* produces a seed capsule. While this seed capsule is still unripe, it can be slit or incised with a sharp knife, and a white, milky exudate will form. This is scraped off, collected into masses (where it turns brown upon air oxidation), and sold to either the licit or the illicit trade as opium.

Opium contains dozens of chemicals, but by far the most important are morphine (approximately 10% by dry weight) and codeine (about 0.5%). Heroin does not exist in nature; it is made by acetylation of morphine. Poppy seed comes from the same plant but contains very, very little narcotic substance. One would have to consume very large quantities of poppy seed to ingest an amount sufficient to be detected by modern tests.

The opium poppy is grown in Southeast Asia; in the area comprising Pakistan, Iran, Afghanistan, and Turkey; and in many other countries. Some of it, of course, enters licit channels that supply our need for morphine and other pain relievers, but the great majority of it is grown to provide morphine, which can be converted illicitly to heroin. An estimated 4 million grams (9000 pounds) of uncut heroin was smuggled into the United States in a recent year. Opium smoking, an ancient habit, is still practiced in some parts of the world, but the big money and trafficking today are in heroin.

Opium is used to prepare camphorated tincture of opium (paregoric), widely used to control diarrhea.

See also NARCOTIC ANALGESICS, OPIATES

OTC. *See* OVER-THE-COUNTER DRUGS

Over-the-Counter Drugs

Over-the-counter drugs and health products are those preparations that can legally be purchased without a prescription in the United States. There are over 300,000 OTC products available, including allergy relief pills, antacids, cold products, dandruff preparations, pregnancy tests, laxatives, antidiarrheals, pain relievers, sleep aids, stay-awake aids, contraceptives, vitamins, weight control products, gas relievers, and wart removers.

OTC drugs should not be used casually; they can be potent medicines with potentially significant side effects. Aspirin, for example, can cause loss of blood in the GI tract and can prolong bleeding time (it should never be used after a tonsillectomy). Extra-strength doses of acetaminophen can cause liver damage. Antihistamines can make one drowsy and ill prepared to operate a car or machinery. Overdoses of antacids can disrupt the normal acid-base balance of the body. Dependence on laxatives is to be deplored, in spite of what the ads would have us believe.

Too much of vitamins A and D is a threat in the human, as these vitamins are toxic in excessive dosage. The phenylpropanolamine (PPA) in nasal decongestants and appetite-suppressant drugs can cause insomnia, restlessness, nausea, and a rise in blood pressure when taken in high doses. Sudafed contains pseudoephedrine, a brain stimulant.

Some OTC products contain 200 mg of caffeine per dose. That is enough to cause muscle tremor and irregular heartbeat in sensitive users, not to mention insomnia. Drug interactions can occur between OTC drugs. Alcohol combined with OTC sleep aids can depress the brain and make you sleepy and ill equipped to drive a car. Antacids can seriously reduce absorption of tetracycline from the intestines.

You would be wise to read the label of every OTC drug you take, for often there are warnings to diabetics, asthmatics, heart patients, automobile drivers, hypertensives, allergy-prone people, and even the healthy person about to use the drug. Recovering alcoholics especially should read labels; some products contain a high percentage of alcohol (NyQuil is 50-proof).

Some drugs sold OTC in Mexico are available only by prescription in the United States. Thus the legal status of an OTC may depend on the country in which it is distributed.

See also individual OTC drugs by name

Oxazepam. *See* TRANQUILIZERS, MINOR

P

Paint Thinner. *See* SOLVENTS AND INHALANTS

Pangamic Acid. *See* "VITAMIN B-15"

Paregoric

Other name: camphorated tincture of opium
Source: compounding
Pharmacology: antidiarrheal
Dose: 1 teaspoonful (5 ml)

The active ingredient in paregoric is morphine. It acts on the intestine to reduce peristalsis and the hyperactivity that is associated with diarrhea. This means that passage of intestinal content slows, there is more time for water to be absorbed, electrolytes are conserved, and in general the diarrhea is relieved. NOTE: Antiperistaltic drugs may worsen the effects of *Shigella*-caused diarrhea.

The antiperistaltic effect of morphine and other opiates is well known. It is what makes heroin addicts chronically constipated.

Paregoric may be obtained on prescription (it's a Schedule III drug). In many states (but not in California) it also is sold OTC in combination with other ingredients as a Schedule V drug, sometimes called an "exempt narcotic." When purchasing paregoric OTC, one must give one's name and address; the pharmacist will keep a record of exempt narcotic sales.

Abuse potential: low. However, we recognize that it is not uncommon for heroin or morphine addicts to acquire a large supply of paregoric when their regular supply of stronger opiate is cut off.

Adverse effects: With the recommended dose of 1 teaspoonful, few if any adverse effects can be expected.

See also DIARRHEA PRODUCTS, OPIUM

Pazo Ointment, Suppositories

Other names for ingredients: benzocaine, ephedrine
Source: compounding
Pharmacology: local anesthetic, vasoconstrictor
Dose: The ointment or the suppository is to be applied or inserted night and morning and after each bowel movement.

The ointment form of this product, sold as a treatment for hemorrhoids, contains benzocaine (local anesthetic), ephedrine (vasoconstrictor), camphor (counterirritant), zinc oxide (protectant), petrolatum (protectant), and lanolin. The suppository form contains the same ingredients except that a vegetable oil is substituted for the petrolatum.

The FDA has concluded that this "shotgun" product lacks evidence of safety and effectiveness in at least 1 ingredient, the combination of ingredients, or the dosage form.

Misuse potential: high. It doesn't make a lot of sense to try to cover up the pain of a serious case of hemorrhoids with a local anesthetic that at best can act only temporarily. A vasoconstrictor, properly applied, might be able to check the bleeding from a minor capillary, but not from a varicose vein. Any serious bleeding should be examined by a physician.

Adverse effects: Self-medication with products containing benzocaine has been known to lead to allergic reactions.

PCP

Other names: phencyclidine, angel dust
Source: illicit synthesis
Pharmacology: complex and unpredictable. Can act as a deliriant, anesthetic, stimulant, depressant, and hallucinogen, seemingly all at the same time.
Dose: 5–10 mg. Found in drug-laced cigarettes, a powder that can be inhaled, or an injectable. Also sold on the street in

liquid form. There is no way of knowing the strength of any street preparation.

What a strange and powerful drug PCP is. At various times it can be a depressant, stimulant, hallucinogen, convulsant, or anesthetic. Regarded by some experts as the single most dangerous drug on the illicit market today, PCP can change people so they will never be normal again. Steve E. Lerner, a San Francisco psychologist and a leading expert on PCP, has compiled clinical information on 1400 PCP users and finds the most prevalent use among white, suburban, affluent youths averaging 14 years at first use. He states that the main problem with PCP is its extreme unpredictability.

PCP (phencyclidine or phenylcyclohexylpiperdine) was marketed by Parke-Davis in 1963 as Sernyl. It was used as an anesthetic, but it produced such strange side effects (incoherent speech, delirium, hallucinations) that its legal use in humans was discontinued in 1965. In 1967 it again appeared, reintroduced by Parke-Davis as an anesthetic called Sernylan, for veterinary use only. PCP is believed to have hit the streets for the first time at the 1967 Monterey Pop Festival. It appeared in San Francisco as the *peace pill* and in 1968 in the East as *hog.* PCP is sold admixed with marijuana, or in variously shaped tablets or capsules. *Angel dust* is a mixture of mint leaves, parsley, or low-grade marijuana laced with PCP. A small packet, weighing about 1.5 g and selling for $10, can be turned into 5 or 10 cigarettes, and 1 such cigarette is all that's needed for a dreamy state that lasts up to 8 hours. The cigarettes are called dusters.

Because PCP is available in liquid form, it can be soaked into ordinary cigarettes or marijuana joints. The products are called Sherms. DAWN data show that PCP ranks seventh in hospital emergency room mentions.

A Los Angeles police officer calls PCP "stronger and more dangerous than LSD." He considers PCP to be the worst of the common psychedelics, for "it produces a void, complete disorientation."

With a low to moderate dose (5–10 mg producing in the adult a 30-to-100-ng/ml blood level), PCP users can show agitation; excitement; gross incoordination; spaced-out, floating euphoria; inability to speak; sweating; and loss of pain sensation leading to stupor, vomiting, hypersalivation, repetitive motor movements, and an eyes-open coma. They may stumble or crawl about (zombie walking). Mentally, this dose of PCP produces distorted images, extreme feelings of apathy, depersonalization, and drowsiness.

Drowsy, intoxicated users of PCP may inexplicably turn violent and irrational, inflicting physical harm on themselves or others. What is more, the strength of PCP-intoxicated persons is described as incredible. One PCP user was able to break open handcuffs locked behind his back. The incredible strength and violent behavior of some PCP users have led police to develop and use the "Taser," an electrical device that can be used at long range to shock the uncontrollable person into submission.

Methods are available for the detection of PCP in the urine of users.

If the PCP trip is such a potential bummer and has such a poor street reputation, why do so many continue to experience it? There are at least four answers:

1. PCP often is deceitfully sold on the street as THC, mescaline, or cocaine. Sometimes it is mixed with LSD. Thus some escapists don't know they are using it.
2. Supplies are plentiful and inexpensive. PCP can be synthesized by amateur chemists using simple equipment and chemicals routinely sold by chemical suppliers. Many suppliers now demand a letterhead on the order, or other proof of legitimate intent, but these precautions can be circumvented.
3. The prospect of a euphoric high from PCP apparently provides enough motivation for users to ignore its traumatic side effects.
4. PCP is inexpensive, makes the user feel good, and, more importantly, makes users with little or no self-esteem feel important.

Hindsight is unfair, but we now know how wise the manufacturer would have been not to have reintroduced PCP after the first marketing established its potential as a psychedelic drug of abuse.

Abuse potential: high

Adverse effects: A mild dose of PCP is 2–5 mg. Marijuana joints have been analyzed that were laced with as much as 75 mg. Overdosage with PCP can produce days-long coma, very high blood pressure, muscular rigidity, and convulsions. Life-support systems and intensive medical management are required to keep the person alive. There is no specific antidote for PCP; the physician can only treat the symptoms—for example, by giving diazepam to control convulsions.

Tolerance to PCP develops, and ever larger doses are required to achieve the desired effects.

After repeated PCP intoxication, users may develop a psychosis not unlike that seen in schizophrenia, and it may be 1 or 2 years before they feel normal again. Users can experience flashbacks, and for a long while they may feel depressed and spaced out. This reaction appears to be due to the storage of the fully psychoactive drug in body fat tissues.

Drug interactions: PCP depresses respiration and heart rate, and its combination with alcohol, another depressant, can trigger an overdose.

Pearls. *See* NITRITES

Pentazocine. *See* TALWIN

Pentothal. *See* BARBITURATES

Pepto-Bismol

Main ingredient: bismuth subsalicylate
Source: compounding
Pharmacology: supposed antidiarrheal
Dose: for adults, either 2 tablespoonfuls of the liquid or 2 tablets

The main ingredient in Pepto-Bismol, bismuth subsalicylate, is a drug that has been around for many years, but we don't have conclusive scientific evidence that it works. In fact, the FDA has prohibited label claims that promise relief of "heartburn and acid indigestion" and has concluded that bismuth salts lack evidence of either safety or effectiveness in treating diarrhea. Consumers Union has advised against the use of Pepto-Bismol liquid.

Most (but not all) of the acute diarrheal attacks we experience will clear up by themselves without the use of any chemical agent. If the diarrhea occurs with a high fever or lasts more than 2 days, see a doctor.

Misuse potential: high

Adverse effects: If you use this product, your tongue and/or stool may turn black (this could obscure fecal darkening due to blood loss). This product contains a salicylate (aspirin is a salicylate), and people who are sensitive to salicylates would want to avoid this product. You can tell if you are ingesting too much aspirin or other salicylate: You will experience ringing in your ears. If this occurs, stop taking the drugs immediately. CAUTION: If you are pregnant or nursing a child, do not take this product without first consulting your physician.

Drug interactions: See your physician before you combine this drug with an oral anticoagulant, or a diabetes or gout drug.

See also DIARRHEA PRODUCTS

Percogesic

Other names of active ingredients: acetaminophen, phenyltoloxamine

Source: synthesis

Pharmacology: pain and fever reliever, antihistamine

Dose: adults and children 12 years and over, 1 or 2 tablets every 4 hours, not to exceed 8 tablets a day; for children 6–12 years, half the adult dose, not to exceed 4 tablets a day.

This product contains acetaminophen in the "standard" dose of 325 mg, plus phenyltoloxamine, an antihistamine. The FDA has warned that antihistamines have no ability to prevent or cure the common cold; they can, however, cause drowsiness and interfere with the operation of a car or machinery.

The manufacturers state that Percogesic is intended for the relief of minor aches and pains of rheumatism and arthritis. However, it is well known that—unlike aspirin—acetaminophen does not possess clinically significant anti-inflammatory activity. True rheumatoid arthritis can be a serious condition requiring the advice of a physician. Acetaminophen clearly is not the drug of choice for rheumatoid arthritis. In fact, masking the pain of the disease without arresting its progress might be worse than no drug at all.

See the section on acetaminophen for the dangers of overdosing, especially with long-term use. Acetaminophen is sold generically for as little as 2.5¢ per tablet. In one store Percogesic sold for $2.49 for 24 tablets, or 4 times as much. Whether you buy acetaminophen generically or by trade name, it is exactly the same drug.

Misuse potential: low to medium. Because of misleading advertising, many people are led to believe that antihistamines can cure the common cold, or hasten recovery. They can do neither. Avoid the use of cold remedies that contain antihistamines.

Adverse effects: If you do not exceed the recommended doses for acetaminophen, you probably will not experience any significant adverse effects. However, excessive doses, especially of the extra-strength preparations, can lead to liver damage. The kidney also is sensitive to overdosage. CAUTION: Persons with a known history of liver disease should avoid excessive use of acetaminophen and should restrict its use to brief periods. WARNING: Antihistamines must be used with considerable caution if you are suffering from peptic ulcer, narrow-angle glaucoma, GI obstruction, enlargement of the prostate gland, or bladder neck obstruction. Most of these adverse effects are due to the anticholinergic properties inherent in many antihistamines. The dry mouth, difficulty in urination, and impotence sometimes seen in antihistamine use are also based on these properties.

Drug interactions: Combining alcohol with acetaminophen can increase the poisonous effects of both on the liver. Either avoid these drug combinations or consult your doctor beforehand. Antihistamine drug interactions are well known. Alcohol combined with antihistamines can cause serious sedation. Barbiturates combined with antihistamines at first cause severe CNS depression; later they nullify each other's actions.

Peyote. *See* MESCALINE

Phenobarbital

Other names: Luminal, Solfoton
Source: synthesis

Pharmacology: mild sedative; anticonvulsant in epilepsy

Dose: as sedative: 15–30 mg (usually 1 or 2 tablets); as anti-convulsant: 100–200 mg (or as individualized)

As a drug, phenobarbital has been used for 75 years and has gained a good reputation as a mild sedative to relieve anxiety and tension and as an effective means of controlling certain types of epileptic seizures.

As described in the section on barbiturates, phenobarbital is a long-acting drug. That means it will require a longer time to take effect, but its effects will last longer than those of, say, Nembutal or Seconal. It also means that phenobarbital is safer to use than one of the fast-acting barbiturates (though certainly not completely safe; the lethal dose of phenobarbital is believed to be about 5 g).

Users of phenobarbital should know that no matter for what purpose taken, this drug will slow down mental and physical reflexes; it is a CNS depressant. Of course, if you are looking for sedation and relief from tension, that is what to expect. But the epileptic patient will have to learn to cope with a possible slower response to stimuli that increases the risk of driving a car or operating machinery.

Phenobarbital is prescribed for use in *grand mal* and psycho-motor types of epilepsy (these are also termed tonic-clonic, and partial seizure, respectively). In epilepsy there is massive, un-controlled discharge of nerve activity from the CNS. Thus a drug such as phenobarbital that depresses CNS activity would be expected to control, but not eliminate, the seizures. The goal is to find the optimum dose of depressant that stops most or all of the attacks but does not oversedate the patient. Phenobarbital is available in timed-release formulations.

Abuse potential: low to medium

Adverse effects: In addition to allergic reactions, phenobarbital can cause idiosyncratic CNS excitement and delirium. It can cause dizziness, mental depression, impaired vision, and a deficiency in red and white blood cells that can lead to fatigue, fever, and sore throat. If any of these symptoms appear, see your doctor. CAUTION: Long-term and/or heavy use of this drug can lead to tolerance and physical dependence involving a serious withdrawal syndrome. Do not abruptly stop taking this drug without first consulting a physician.

Drug interactions: See the section on barbiturates. Phenobarbital combined with Dilantin can cause either an increased or a decreased Dilantin blood level. Combining alcohol with any barbiturate is inviting tragedy from synergistic depression of respiration. You can fall asleep and stop breathing in your sleep. Combining phenobarbital with a tranquilizer, opiate, or any other CNS depressant can cause oversedation. Allergic reactions to barbiturates are known; they consist of skin rash, swelling, or fever. Report any untoward effects to your physician immediately. In nursing mothers this drug will appear in breast milk.

See also BARBITURATES

Phenylcyclidine. *See* PCP

Phenylephrine. *See* COLD REMEDIES

Phenylpropanolamine

Other names: PPA, Propadrine
Source: synthesis
Pharmacology: decongestant, appetite suppressant, sympathomimetic
Dose: variable, but in the range of 9.4–75 mg in various OTC products

NOTE: Phenylpropanolamine is found in many OTC products, including Acutrim, Alka-Seltzer Plus, Allerest, Appedrine, Bayer Children's Cold Tablets and Cough Syrup, Cheracol Plus, Children's CoTylenol Chewable, Children's Hold, Comtrex, Congesprin, Contac, Coricidin, Creamacoat, Daycare, Dexatrim, Dorcol, Dristan, Formula 44D, 4-Way, Halls Metho-Lyptus, Pertussin, Pyrroxate, Robitussin-CF, St. Joseph Cold Tablet, Sinarest, Sine-Off Extra, Spec-T Sore, Sucrets, Triaminic, Trind, and Tussagesic.

PPA is a sympathomimetic. That means it is pharmacologically related to adrenaline and would be expected to produce similar actions in the body. One of these actions, its ability to constrict blood vessels, is the basis for its wide use as a nasal decongestant. When applied locally, PPA can relieve the nasal stuffiness of colds and allergies by constricting blood vessels in the mucous membranes of the nose. This shrinkage improves nasal breathing, promotes drainage, and relieves the stuffiness. Nasal decongestants such as PPA can be taken orally, too, but their effects are less intense than when applied topically and locally.

Some users of nasal decongestants experience a *rebound* congestive effect in which nasal stuffiness is even worse after the drug's effects wear off. This rebound necessitates taking another dose of shrinker, and then another, until the person is sniffing the inhaler all day long, but with no real long-lasting relief. This type of drug dependence is termed *functional dependence.*

The use of PPA as a diet aid is discussed under appetite-suppressant drugs. WARNING: Do not exceed the recommended dosage of PPA. If you have high blood pressure, check with your physician before using any PPA product.

Misuse potential: medium

Adverse effects: No matter how taken, sympathomimetic decongestants get into the bloodstream and exert their effects on the brain, heart, and blood pressure. Although it is true that PPA was designed to have minimal side effects, it can stimulate the heart and brain, and some users may discover their heart beating at a faster rate, or their mind stimulated at bedtime after using PPA as a decongestant. Those at risk if they use PPA are heart disease patients, hypertensives, hyperthyroid patients, those using digitalis, and persons with glaucoma or those who have difficulty emptying their bladder.

According to the Center for Science in the Public Interest, there is overwhelming evidence that PPA is a dangerous drug. The Center states that PPA can cause high blood pressure and brain seizures. This is disputed by the PPA pill manufacturers.

Drug interactions: Taken concurrently with other sympathomimetics (such as epinephrine) or with ergot alkaloids, PPA can cause excessive stimulation of the heart, leading to rapid pulse and high blood pressure. PPA counteracts the action of antihypertensive drugs. Irregular heartbeat can occur if PPA and digitalis are combined. The use of any monoamine oxidase inhibitor drug simultaneously with PPA is strongly contraindicated because of the possibility of dangerously high blood pressure.

See also APPETITE-SUPPRESSANT DRUGS, COLD REMEDIES, LOOK-ALIKES

Placebo

A placebo is an inactive, sham drug that is given (1) to satisfy a demanding patient, or (2) to test whether a drug response is real or based upon expectations.

A patient may be given a placebo that looks exactly like his or her real medication (which the person thinks he or she needs to stay well) but that contains nothing more active than milk sugar. The patient thinks that he or she is getting the real drug and is satisfied.

Before a new drug can enter the marketplace, it is tested "placebo-double blind." This means that half of the test patients receive milk sugar and half the real thing. Neither the patients nor the administering nurse know who is receiving which (that's the double-blind part). If the placebo-takers say they get as much relief as the real-drug-takers, one can conclude that the drug does not have much of an action of its own.

People respond to placebos because they *believe* they are receiving a real drug, and therefore they *expect* to get a result. *Because* they expect a result, they get it. That's termed the placebo effect. It is a matter of mind controlling body response. Consider this example: In one study of a new tranquilizer, 40% of the patients who received the placebo said it worked and made them feel better. In another study on pain, it was discovered that the placebo satisfactorily relieved pain of various causes in 35% of patients. By comparison, in the same study, large doses of morphine relieved pain in only 75% of the subjects. This result shows that placebos can have great power in the human that must be taken into account in evaluating a drug's effectiveness. Many other examples of placebo response have been reported in medical literature, including the successful application of placebos in the treatment of arthritis, hay fever, hypertension, headache, constipation, acne, seasickness, ulcers, and even warts. Placebos can even induce typical drug side effects such as skin rash, nausea, and anaphylactic shock.

In a British study, aspirin tablets with a brand name marking were found to be more effective in relieving headache than unbranded aspirin, apparently because the patients believed, from past experience, advertising, and hearsay, that they could trust the branded tablets to be effective.

The placebo effect is but one manifestation of the more profound observation that the mind and the body are inseparable and that the human organism has a great capacity for self-healing. Hence, attempts to treat most bodily diseases as though the mind were in no way involved must be considered archaic. Seventy-five years ago, Sir William Osler, the father of modern medicine, said, "The cure of tuberculosis depends more on what the patient has in his head than what he has in his chest." Research today supports the view that almost every ill that can befall the body—from headache to heart disease—can be influenced in some way by the person's mental state.

Researchers today are investigating the theory that good mental attitudes can fight off disease. They find support for this idea in the knowledge that white blood cell activity is affected by certain neurotransmitters in the body. There is also evidence that the immune system may influence the nervous system.

As a consumer of drugs, you should know that the relief you get from a drug preparation might possibly be due to the placebo effect. You might be getting relief because you expect to get it and want to get it. This knowledge should make you cautious about any new, untried, or highly touted drug that is advertised as working wonders.

Placidyl

Other name: ethchlorvynol
Source: synthesis
Pharmacology: oral hypnotic (sleep-inducer)
Dose: Adults: 500 mg taken orally at bedtime; may be increased to 750 mg for users who fail to respond to 500 mg. Maximum single dose is 1000 mg. Placidyl comes in 200- and 500-mg red capsules and a 750-mg green capsule.

Placidyl is not a barbiturate, but along with Noludar, Valium, and Doriden, it is similar in pharmacological properties to the barbiturates. All of these drugs are sleep-inducers that have been prescribed in place of the more dangerous barbiturates. Placidyl, introduced in 1955, acts to induce sleep in 15 minutes to 1 hour, and its effects last for 5 hours.

The danger with Placidyl, as with so many sleep-inducing agents, lies in the great temptation to use, reuse, and finally overrely. It is just too easy to get to depend upon a chemical for sleep. And with Placidyl, there is a real risk of developing a dependency, either physical or psychological, with a significant withdrawal syndrome when the drug is finally discontinued. People who have a history of mental depression or alcohol or drug dependence probably should not be given Placidyl. In any event, do not use this drug for more than 7 days; preferably use it only once or twice occasionally if you must.

Abuse potential: medium

Adverse effects: Users have reported the following adverse effects, in decreasing order of severity; allergic reactions, including rash, jaundice, and itching; one type of low-white-blood-cell count; nausea, vomiting, and gastric upset; dizziness and facial numbness; and blurred vision.

Pregnancy category C; there is evidence that this drug might cause birth defects and therefore should be avoided during pregnancy. CAUTION: It is risky to operate a car or machinery while under the influence of this drug. Poisoning from overdosage of Placidyl is characterized by severe depression of respiration, deep coma, low blood pressure, slow heart rate, and low body temperature.

Drug interactions: Strictly avoid the combined use of alcohol and Placidyl, for dangerous oversedation of the brain may occur. The same is true for the combination of Placidyl with barbiturates, tranquilizers, or monoamine oxidase inhibitors. Placidyl can speed up the body's metabolism of coumarin-type anticoagulants, necessitating a change in dose of the latter. Concurrent use of Placidyl and tricyclic antidepressants such as Elavil may result in delirium.

See also SLEEP AIDS

Poppers. *See* NITRITES

Poppy Seed. *See* OPIUM

Pramoxine

Other names: Tronolane Anesthetic Cream for Hemorrhoids, Tronolane Anesthetic Suppositories for Hemorrhoids, proctoFoam non-steroid

Source: compounding
Pharmacology: local anesthetic
Dose: apply up to 5 times daily

Pramoxine is the generic name for a topical (local) anesthetic sold OTC as Tronolane Anesthetic Cream for Hemorrhoids, Tronolane Anesthetic Suppositories for Hemorrhoids, and as proctoFoam/non-steroid spray foam. Promoted for the relief of the burning and itching of hemorrhoids, this topical anesthetic is chemically different from the benzocaine type and therefore should not be expected to cause the allergic reactions of the "caine" products. This does not mean, however, that hypersensitivity to pramoxine will never occur in any patient.

Hemorrhoid patients who use topical anesthetics should know that temporary relief of pain does not necessarily mean that healing has occurred. Local anesthetics dull the nerves; they don't heal. If you have bleeding, or if the hemorrhoid condition persists, see a physician. Do not try to mask your symptoms by prolonged use of this or any other anesthetic.

Misuse potential: low

Adverse effects: Pramoxine has a low sensitizing index, with few toxic reactions. Do not get this product into your eyes. If you have bleeding, see a physician.

Pregnancy Categories

The FDA has established a system for rating the safety of drugs used during pregnancy. Teratogens—drugs that can cause birth defects—must be assiduously avoided during pregnancy, and pregnant women need guidelines in drug-taking. If it is an elective drug (for headache, sleep, acne, anxiety), the choice to avoid may be easy. But if the drug is needed for infection, arrhythmia, epilepsy, blood clot, hypertension, migraine, psoriasis, or depression, the decision to use or not can be difficult.

Women can check with their physician or pharmacist to determine in which of the five pregnancy categories a drug is listed: A, B, C, D, or X. The A category is the safest, and the X category is the most dangerous. Here is the breakdown of FDA Pregnancy Categories for teratogenicity:

- Category A. The safest drug category for use in pregnancy. Studies in pregnant women reveal no potential for causing birth defects.
- Category B. Either there is no evidence of teratogenicity from animal tests, with no available concurrent data from studies in pregnant women, or there is evidence of teratogenicity in animal tests but negative results on birth defects from studies in pregnant women. The risk of using this drug is minimal.
- Category C. Either there is evidence of teratogenicity from animal tests but no concurrent available data from studies in pregnant women, or there simply are no data from either animal or human studies. There is a risk in taking these drugs, and the patient and her doctor must decide.
- Category D. Studies in pregnant women reveal clear evidence of teratogenicity. Use is contraindicated in all cases except possibly life-threatening situations where alternate drugs are of no use.
- Category X. Avoid at all costs. Clear evidence of birth defects from animal or human studies.

Some older drugs apparently have not been categorized. If information is unavailable, the best decision is to avoid the drug during pregnancy. Alcohol is a potent teratogen, but it is not rated because it does not come under the jurisdiction of the FDA. (Alcohol and tobacco are regulated by another federal agency.)

See also TERATOGENS

Premarin

Other name: Conjugated Estrogen Tablets, USP
Source: pregnant mares' urine
Pharmacology: female sex hormone
Dose: Premarin is administered in many different ways. It is given regularly or cyclically (3 weeks on and 1 week off), for vasomotor symptoms (1.25 mg daily), for atrophic vaginitis and kraurosis vulvae (0.3–1.25 mg or more daily), for female hypogonadism (2.5–7.5 mg daily for 20 days followed by a 10-day rest), for female castration and primary ovarian failure (1.25 mg

daily, cyclically), and for osteoporosis (0.625 mg daily, cyclically). Follow your physician's directions exactly.

When women enter the menopause (change of life), typically at ages 45–52, their ovaries begin to cease the production of female sex hormones. Cessation of estrogen production can—in the worst cases—result in nervousness, hot flashes, chills, excitability, crying spells, insomnia, urinary frequency, and a vaginitis that interferes with sexual intercourse. Many of these symptoms can be anticipated by premenstrual counseling, but others (especially those involving the vascular system) may require prescribed estrogen.

Premarin is one of the most highly prescribed estrogens for use in menopausal women. It is prescribed for vaginitis and to retard progression of estrogen-deficiency-produced osteoporosis (when used with other measures such as diet and exercise). Premarin is obtained from pregnant mares' urine and contains equilin and dihydroequilin (two horse sex hormones) and estrone (a human estrogen). Equine estrogens are similar enough to function in humans.

There is no doubt that estrogens are helpful in treating symptoms of the menopause, but they must not be overrelied on or used for too long a time. Caution is required because of studies in laboratory animals that indicate that long-term, continuous use of estrogen increases the risk of cancer of the cervix, vagina, breast, and liver. While at present there is no convincing evidence that the same will occur in the human, there is need for caution, especially in women with a family history of breast cancer. We do know that there is a statistical link between cancer of the lining of the uterus (womb) and the continuous use of prescribed estrogen for more than 1 year. Further, there is evidence of a twofold to threefold increase in the risk of gallbladder disease in women receiving estrogen for menopausal symptoms. For all of these reasons and others, the FDA now recommends only short-term use of estrogens in the menopause, and at the lowest dose needed to relieve the symptoms. Premarin for treatment of osteoporosis is far longer-term.

WARNING: Estrogens should not be used during pregnancy, even for a day.

Misuse potential: low

Adverse effects: Users have reported the following adverse

effects with estrogenic drugs: breakthrough bleeding, dysmenorrhea, amenorrhea during and after treatment, vaginal candidiasis, breast tenderness, nausea, vomiting, cramps, jaundice,
discoloration of the skin, loss of scalp hair, intolerance to contact
lenses, headache, dizziness, and mental depression.

Drug interactions: Estrogens may combine with aminoca-
prioc acid adversely to increase the chance of blood clotting.
There is some evidence that diabetics should take estrogen only
with caution. Phenobarbital has been shown to increase the
body's metabolism of estrogen. Combining estrogen with hy-
drocortisone can result in excessive corticosteroid effects. Patients taking estrogen should avoid taking excessive amounts of
mineral oil, as the oil could impair absorption of the estrogens.
Rifampin may speed up the metabolism of estrogen.

See also ESTROGENS

Preparation H

Ingredients: shark liver oil, live yeast cell derivative
Source: compounding
Pharmacology: advertised as a treatment for hemorrhoids
Dose: The ointment or suppository is used night and morn-
ing or whenever the need arises.

This expensive, widely advertised treatment for hemorrhoids
holds over 50% of the market and has sales in excess of $60
million yearly. Yet it contains ingredients the experts say don't
work. Preparation H contains shark liver oil (3%) and live yeast
cell derivative. Live yeast cell derivative is without evidence of
effectiveness for any anorectal use. Shark liver oil does not show
evidence of being a safe and effective wound-healing drug,
although it is an effective protectant if used in 50% or greater
concentrations.

Preparation H, despite its popularity and high cost, is not
recognized by the FDA as safe and effective in the treatment
of hemorrhoids, based upon at least 1 ingredient, the combination of ingredients, or the dosage form. There is no acceptable
evidence that Preparation H can shrink hemorrhoids, reduce
inflammation, or heal injured tissue. There is evidence that you
are wasting your money on this product.

See also HEMORRHOIDAL PRODUCTS

ProctoFoam. *See* PRAMOXINE

Prolamine Maximum Strength Capsules

Other name of active ingredient: phenylpropanolamine
Source: synthesis
Pharmacology: appetite suppressant
Dose: 1 capsule (37.5 mg) at 10:00 A.M. and at 4:00 P.M., with a glassful of water

One of the ways the ads tell you that you can control weight is through the use of drugs that stimulate your brain and put you into an excited state in which you have no interest in food. Phenylpropanolamine is a stimulant to the brain and heart. In the hefty dose of 37.5 mg twice daily it will put you into an artificial state of excitement, and you probably will feel less like eating. However, if you decide to rely on a drug to reduce your appetite, you are going to have to keep taking the drug for as long as you want to keep off weight. That might mean that you are stimulated night and day for weeks or months. Such artificial excitement creates a strain on all but the healthiest bodies. You might discover that your heart is beating rapidly all day long, or that you simply cannot get to sleep at night. And usually, when use of the drug is stopped, weight is quickly regained. How much wiser it is to recognize that restricted food intake and/or increase in physical activity are the only sensible ways to accomplish weight control. The motivation for that must come from within, not from a bottle.

Misuse potential: high

Adverse effects: Phenylpropanolamine is a sympathomimetic (see that section) and has the potential for all the adverse effects associated with these stimulants. Users of phenylpropanolamine have reported headache, rapid heartbeat, irregular heartbeat, dizziness, nervousness, insomnia, and agitation. CAUTION: Unless approved by your physician, do not give this product to children under 12 years of age or to anyone suffering from high blood pressure, diabetes, or heart, kidney, or thyroid disease. Pregnant or nursing women or anyone over 60 years should not use this product.

Drug interactions: Do not combine this product with any

other brain stimulant or nasal decongestant, including ephedrine or epinephrine, as dangerously high blood pressure may result. Phenylpropanolamine will nullify the effects of drugs taken to relieve high blood pressure. Never combine this product with a monoamine oxidase inhibitor drug such as Parnate or Nardil because of the possibility of excessive brain and heart stimulation.

See also SYMPATHOMIMETICS, PHENYLPROPANOLAMINE

Pseudoephedrine

Other names: found in dozens of products; see discussion
Source: synthesis
Pharmacology: nasal decongestant, bronchodilator, sympathomimetic
Dose: Adult, typically 30–60 mg (1 tablet in most products). Do not exceed 240 mg in 24 hours.

When two chemical compounds differ from each other not in structure but in the way their bonds are arranged in space, they are said to be stereoisomers of each other. Pseudoephedrine is a stereoisomer of ephedrine, and differs from it enough to have only one fifth the blood-pressure-raising power of ephedrine. Pseudoephedrine also is less active in stimulating the CNS.

Pseudoephedrine works by stimulating nerve endings to release norepinephrine, which in turn stimulates blood vessels throughout the body to contract, but especially blood vessels of the upper respiratory tract. Constriction of blood vessels in the nose helps shrink swollen and inflamed membranes, too. This is the basis for the use of pseudoephedrine as a nasal decongestant. Other commonly used decongestants are phenylpropanolamine and phenylephrine.

Pseudoephedrine is found in dozens of prescription-only and OTC products as a nasal decongestant, usually in 30-to-60-mg doses. A few of the prescription-only products containing pseudoephedrine are: Actifed with Codeine, Dimetane-DX Cough Syrup, Fedahist, Novafed, and Novahistine Expectorant. A few of the OTC products containing pseudoephedrine are Benadryl Decongestant, Chlortrimeton Decongestant, Contac Capsules, CoTylenol Cold Medication, Dristan Ultra, Neo-Synephrinol, Robitussin-PE, Sine-Aid, Sinutab Maximum Strength, Sudafed, and Tylenol Sinus Medication Maximum Strength.

Note that many of these OTC products are of the "shotgun" variety in which the user is forced to experience the side effects or possible adverse effects of all of the ingredients to get the benefit of only one. The FDA is highly critical of shotgun products.

Misuse potential: medium

Adverse effects: While pseudoephedrine, a sympathomimetic, does not have the brain and blood pressure stimulatory effects of drugs such as epinephrine, it can cause a rise in heart rate and blood pressure and stimulation of the brain leading to insomnia, especially in sensitive users. CAUTION: Pseudoephedrine should be used only with the advice of your physician if you are suffering from high blood pressure, heart disease, diabetes, or a sensitivity to ephedrine. Pseudoephedrine can cause restlessness, insomnia, and dryness of the mouth and throat. Long-term use of any nasal shrinker is to be avoided. CAUTION: Some OTC products contain unusually high doses of pseudoephedrine, considering their use. Rondec Oral Drops for *infants* contain 25 mg of pseudoephedrine per milliliter; the indicated dose for a 9–18-month-old infant is 1 ml. Contrast that with a 60-mg dose indicated for a grown man. People over 60 years are more likely to have adverse reactions to any sympathomimetic. Overdosage in this age group has been reported to cause convulsions, hallucinations, CNS depression, and death.

Drug interactions: Simultaneous use of pseudoephedrine and monoamine oxidase inhibitors such as Parnate or Nardil can result in a serious hypertensive crisis in which blood pressure rises dangerously and the brain is stimulated. Pseudoephedrine can increase blood levels of glucose and thus interfere with insulin requirements; it also can reduce the antihypertensive effects of methyldopa and reserpine.

See also COLD REMEDIES, SYMPATHOMIMETICS

Psilocybin. *See* MUSHROOMS

Psychedelics

In 1956, H. Osmond coined the term *psychedelics* to refer to drugs that "expand" the mind. He wrote, "A psychedelic compound is one like LSD or mescaline which enriches the mind and enlarges the vision. It is this kind of experience which promotes the greatest possibility for examining those areas most interesting to psychiatry. . . ." Osmond intended that the term "psychedelic" emphasize the nonpsychotic actions of these psychotropic agents.

In loose usage *psychedelic* has come to mean about the same as hallucinogen, but as Osmond intended, there is a difference. The term *psychotomimetic* comes closer to describing LSD's hallucinogenic-model psychosis effects.

All of the psychedelics sold on the street are Schedule I controlled substances (see section on controlled substances). They are considered to be high-abuse-potential drugs that certain people are tempted to use to "expand the mind," gain religious insight, or just experiment with. But whenever they are used, there is the possibility of the drug triggering a "bummer" trip or in rare instances a psychotic breakdown. Also, one has no idea of what drug one is actually getting in a street sale.

See also HALLUCINOGEN

Q

Quaalude. *See* METHAQUALONE

Quackery

Quackery is the promotion and sale of useless remedies promising relief from health conditions. Quackery is a $10 billion-a-year business in America. Three areas in which quackery flourishes are cancer, arthritis, and aging. The modern quack's prime target is the senior citizen; the approaches include the illustrated brochure, the supermarket press, TV commercials, testimonial ads, storefront clinics, and phony foundations. Among older persons, 80% have at least 1 chronic health condition. The quack feeds on ignorance. An FDA study found that three quarters of people in a survey believed that extra vitamins provide more pep and energy; one fifth thought that diseases such as cancer and arthritis are caused by vitamin and mineral deficiencies; and 12% surveyed reported self-diagnosed arthritis, rheumatism, or heart trouble.

Hundreds of phony diets, drugs, devices, and therapies have been promoted as cures for cancer, including jojoba oil, goat serum, Hett cancer serum, antineol, Bamfolin, CH-23, H.11, Polonine, the grape diet, the Gerson diet, the macrobiotic diet, the Rand treatment, and the Chase dietary method (including daily enemas with lemon juice, grapefruit juice, or coffee: a "poison by mouth but a stimulant rectally").

Dozens of drugs and worthless products have been sold as treatments or cures of arthritis, including ginseng, aloe vera, cocaine, Novocain, Gerovial H-3, DMSO, Flagyl, Mericin, Defecin, Norkon, DPA, Doxyhydren, bee venom, Honegar, and alfalfa seed. All of these have been rejected by the FDA as worthless against arthritis.

Cancer quackery has fleeced thousands of Americans of millions of dollars. The cancer patient is especially vulnerable and will place his trust in almost any "cure" that is proffered by even the most unscrupulous dealer. President Taft once said, "There are none so credulous as sufferers from disease," and this is especially true of the frightened victims of cancer.

Today Americans are trying to make up their minds about Laetrile, a substance obtained from apricot, peach, or bitter almond kernels and strongly supported by well-organized groups across the country. The FDA has already branded it worthless, and worse, for the vain hope it holds out to cancer victims keeps them from seeking help from qualified sources. Laetrile's supporters call it vitamin B_{17}; their most recent claim is that cancer is a vitamin B_{17} deficiency disease and that therefore Laetrile is needed to prevent as well as treat cancer. Key aspects of the drive in support of Laetrile are (1) attempts to discredit the medical establishment and (2) attempts to elevate Laetrile's status by offering scientific or pseudoscientific explanations of how it works to cure cancer. The "active ingredient" in Laetrile is not new; it has been listed in chemistry reference books for a long time as amygdalin, a substance that in no way fits our modern definition of a vitamin. Amygdalin is potentially toxic, since it contains a cyanide group (cyanide is used in gas-death chambers), and there are verified reports of poisonings when individuals have consumed too many apricot kernels. In one case, a 10-month-old child died from swallowing a number of her father's Laetrile pills. Analysis confirmed a high level of cyanide in her blood.

Amygdalin (Laetrile), says the FDA, has never been found to have any anticancer activity when tested in animals. Laetrile is, in fact, one of the most thoroughly tested cancer "cures." It has been investigated by the California Department of Public Health, Canadian authorities, 4 independent cancer research centers, and the National Cancer Institute (which tested Laetrile on 5 separate occasions between 1957 and 1975). No established drug firm has backed Laetrile. According to the final report of a federally sponsored clinical trial of the efficacy of Laetrile in conjunction with vitamin supplements and the special diets advocated by those who claim that the substance is an effective cancer treatment, Laetrile "is of no substantive value in the treatment of cancer." Of the 156 patients treated with the substance, only 5 showed any improvement for a period of more than 2 months, and they subsequently became more ill.

Laetrile has been banned by the federal government because the FDA has not approved a new drug application (NDA) from its sponsors, due to inadequate scientific proof of its safety and effectiveness as a drug. In 1979 the U.S. Supreme Court ruled unanimously that the Food, Drug, and Cosmetic Act allows no exceptions to its safety and effectiveness provisions and that the FDA can thus legally ban the interstate shipment of Laetrile. Attempts to market Laetrile as a food supplement have also been denied.

We must be vigilant, cautious, and suspicious to escape the onslaught of deceitful advertising all around us. Even today we read ads for magnetic bracelets, Royal jelly rejuvenation cream, Sauna arm belts, Amphenol Diet Pills, Stud capsules, Bio Calendar Health System, Full and Firm Bust Developer, Full Stop Slim Cubes, Bio Derm 21 (wrinkle cream), Le Grande Big Bosom Creme, Active hair grower, Japanese erection ring, Stay Hard Guardian, and Instant Stimu Cream. (All of these ads actually appeared and were the bases of FDA legal action.)

Besides the brazen quackery, there are the more subtle, so-phisticated, half-truth ads for colon cleaners, diet aids, and vitamins that will give you more energy. Buyer, beware!

See also ALOE VERA, "VITAMIN B-15"

R

Reye Syndrome

A statistical link has been established between aspirin and Reye syndrome (pronounced "Rye"), a life-threatening condition that may follow influenza or chicken pox in children (including teenagers). Reye syndrome (RS) is characterized by sudden vomiting, violent headaches, and unusual behavior in children who appear to be recovering from an often mild viral illness. Fatal in about one quarter of cases, RS was named after an Australian pathologist who in 1963 accurately described it as an edema (swelling) of the brain combined with liver malfunction. Data from four studies statistically link the use of salicylates during the antecedent viral illness with the development of Reye syndrome. The data are inconclusive (and are disputed by aspirin manufacturers), but nonetheless the FDA has urged patients not to use aspirin to treat their children's chicken-pox flulike symptoms and has ordered that all aspirin packages carry such a warning. Acetaminophen, certain antibiotics, and certain antiemetics have been used just prior to the onset of symptoms of Reye syndrome. Although the connection is even more tenuous than with aspirin, there is the possibility that these drugs, too, contribute to or affect the course of the syndrome, and should therefore be avoided in children with flulike infections, measles, or chicken pox.

Until we have more information about the pathogenesis of Reye syndrome and the role of salicylate in it, prudence dictates that aspirin in any form should be given to children suffering from the flu or chicken pox only on direct advice of the family physician.

See also ASPIRIN, TIGAN

Ritalin

Other name: methylphenidate
Source: synthesis
Pharmacology: mild CNS stimulant
Dose: individualized. Adults, usually 20–30 mg daily in divided doses 2–3 times daily 30–45 minutes before meals. In children 6 years and older Ritalin should be started in small doses with possible weekly increases. Ritalin is dispensed in 5-, 10-, and 20-mg tablets.

Strictly speaking, methylphenidate is not an amphetamine, although, like them, it has a CNS-stimulatory action; it has less dramatic effects upon respiration and blood pressure. It has been used since 1956 and is recognized in the *United States Pharmacopoeia.*

Ritalin is a very well known drug because of its use in children suffering from attention-deficit disorders (previously termed minimal brain dysfunction, or hyperkinetic-child syndrome). These children typically are hyperactive, have short attention spans, are emotional and impulsive, and can be disruptive in the classroom. Some of them are so hyperactive they cannot even sit down to eat a meal. Paradoxically, some of these children calm down when given Ritalin, a CNS stimulant. The mechanism by which Ritalin works to accomplish its calming action is unknown. It is not to be used in children under 6 years.

Ritalin also is used to treat narcolepsy patients—people suffering from an uncontrollable desire to fall asleep, and who may do so as often as 50 times a day. This debilitating sleep disorder afflicts more than 200,000 Americans. The sleep episodes are brief, may be precipitated by emotional situations, and can occur even when standing up or talking.

Misuse potential: low. There has been criticism of the use of Ritalin in children who have not been properly evaluated or diagnosed and to whom the drug is given indiscriminately with the hope it might work.

Adverse effects: CAUTION: Methylphenidate (Ritalin)

should be used with caution in patients who have a history of alcoholism or drug dependence, because tolerance and physical dependence can easily develop, and withdrawal can lead to severe depression. Pregnant women should consult with their physician before taking this drug. Additional adverse effects that have been reported by some users include nervousness and insomnia; allergies, including skin rash and fever; rapid heart rate with possible arrhythmia; nausea; and dizziness.

Drug interactions: Methylphenidate appears to inhibit the body's destruction of tricyclic antidepressants; thus their serum levels may increase significantly. Concomitant use of methylphenidate and guanethidine may interfere with the control of high blood pressure; this combination should be avoided. Methylphenidate, because of its similarity to the amphetamines, should not be given in combination with monoamine oxidase inhibitors or any pressor agent because dangerously high blood pressure may result. Methylphenidate may inhibit the body's metabolism of anticonvulsants such as Dilantin, necessitating a reduction in dosage of these agents.

See also AMPHETAMINES

Rolaids. *See* ANTACIDS

S

Salicylates

Any drug or chemical that is a derivative of salicylic acid, $C_7H_6O_3$, can be regarded as a salicylate. Aspirin (acetylsalicylic acid), of course, is a salicylate, as are salicylamide, magnesium salicylate, triethanolamine salicylate, oil of wintergreen (methyl salicylate), and sodium salicylate. Aspirin is discussed in its own section.

Salicylamide is not considered to be an effective remedy for pain, fever, and inflammation at low doses and is considered to be too toxic at higher doses. The FDA says that salicylamide is not a safe and effective drug. It should not be used.

Salicylic acid itself is widely available, but not for treating pain or fever. It is used in creams, ointments, and shampoos for removal of corns, calluses, and warts, as a skin cleanser, and as a treatment for acne, psoriasis, athlete's foot, and dandruff. Salicylic acid accomplishes all these actions because of its keratolytic power (it destroys the outer layers of the skin). CAUTION: Do not apply salicylic acid to the face, genitals, or on mucous membranes. Diabetics should not use salicylic acid because of their poor healing powers.

Oil of wintergreen (the methyl ester of salicylic acid) is a liquid salicylate with a pleasant odor; it can be absorbed through the skin and can enter the general circulation by this route. There have been systemic poisonings when too much of it was applied to large skin areas. Oil of wintergreen is employed as a counterirritant in the form of salves and ointments. See the section on counterirritants.

A surprisingly large number of people are allergic to aspirin and other salicylates; in some, life can be threatened by the allergic response. See the section on aspirin.

Salicylates are excreted in the breast milk of nursing mothers. If applied to large skin areas, overabsorption of salicylates can occur; symptoms of poisoning include vomiting, nausea, or ringing in the ears.

See also ASPIRIN, COUNTERIRRITANTS

Scheduled Drug. *See* CONTROLLED SUBSTANCES

Scopolamine

Other names: belladonna alkaloid, hyoscine

Sources: solanaceous plants such as *Atropa belladonna, Hyoscyamus niger,* and *Datura* species

Pharmacology: anticholinergic, antiemetic, antimotion sickness

Dose: less than 1 mg

Scopolamine acts as an anticholinergic drug—that is, it antagonizes the actions of the neurotransmitter acetylcholine and depresses the parasympathetic nervous system. Its actions are quite similar to those of atropine except for the CNS, where atropine stimulates but scopolamine in low doses acts as a sedative.

For treating motion sickness, scopolamine is available on prescription as Transderm-Scop, a skin patch that will deliver scopolamine to the skin for absorption into the blood.

Scopolamine combined with morphine can induce a semiconscious state in which the patient does not remember events that take place. This temporary amnesia is called "twilight sleep" and has been used in obstetrics to cause loss of memory about events during labor or surgery. In large enough doses scopolamine can be used to induce sleep. But the OTC sleep preparations containing scopolamine contain only a tiny dose of the drug.

Scopolamine dilates the pupil of the eye (mydriasis) and paralyzes accommodation (cyclopegia).

Adverse effects: Scopolamine has a great potential to produce confusion and even delirium, especially in elderly patients. In high doses, it can be life threatening. Symptoms of scopolamine poisoning include speech and motor disturbances, nausea and vomiting, and delirium.

Abuse potential: low

Drug interaction: Watch for overdepression of the CNS when scopolamine is combined with alcohol or other CNS depressants. Combine scopolamine with other anticholinergics or with antihistamines only with care.

See also ATROPINE, JIMSONWEED

Seconal

Other names: secobarbital sodium, "reds"
Source: synthesis
Pharmacology: hypnotic (sleeping pill); CNS depressant
Dose: Individualized. Usually 100 mg at bedtime. The aged or debilitated typically receive less. Seconal is available in red 50- and 100-mg capsules.

Seconal is a barbiturate—that is, a derivative of barbituric acid. Barbiturates are discussed in their own section.

The CNS-depressant action of Seconal is the basis for its use as a hypnotic in the treatment of insomnia. It is far better not to use any drug to treat insomnia, but in certain very difficult cases drugs appear to be the only way to sleep. Barbiturates are very effective sleep-inducers. Seconal and the other rapid-acting barbiturates usually act in 30 minutes, give a refreshing night's sleep, and leave one feeling reasonably well the next morning. However, barbiturates depress the amount of time spent in REM sleep, and this is undesirable, for dreaming is considered a valuable psychotherapeutic purge. Barbiturates are not pain relievers at the usual dose.

One major problem with Seconal and the other barbiturates is their ability to depress the reflex that controls respiration. If enough is given, breathing will stop. And if alcohol is also present, it will stop all too easily. Another problem with all barbiturates is development of tolerance and possible physical dependence. Seconal appears to lose its effectiveness by the end of 2 weeks of continual use. This prompts the user to increase the dose again and again, until prodigious quantities are taken each day. Physical addiction is too often the result, and if the user quits cold turkey, the withdrawal syndrome that can occur can involve convulsions and be life-threatening.

The explanation for the development of tolerance lies in Seconal's ability to induce the formation of liver enzymes that catalyze the biotransformation of Seconal. The more drug in the blood, the greater the liver's synthesis of transforming enzymes. If the drug is removed, the enzyme levels will fall, but while they are still high they can cross over and catalyze the metabolism of many other substances.

These two side effects—depression of respiration and induction of liver enzymes—make barbiturates among the worst choices of drugs for inducing sleep.

Abuse potential: high. Seconal is a common street drug. It is taken orally or by injection, alone or in combination with an opiate (a dangerous mixture, since both are potent respiratory depressants). Doctors should take care not to prescribe large numbers of Seconal to any one patient, and patients should never keep large numbers of doses around the house. Sometimes barbiturates are stolen from medicine cabinets.

Adverse effects: Users have reported unnatural drowsiness, confusion, nightmares (when the drug is removed), anxiety, hallucinations, depressed breathing, nausea, vomiting, a too-slow heart, low blood pressure, fainting, and allergic reactions.

WARNING: Seconal and other barbiturates are high-abuse-potential drugs; they can lead to tolerance and physical addiction. Use only sparingly and occasionally, if you must use them at all. Seconal is a Schedule II drug.

Drug interactions: WARNING: Combining alcohol with Seconal can lead to fatal respiratory depression; the two drugs act synergistically. Because of its enzyme-inducing actions, Seconal speeds up the body's breakdown of many other drugs, including methoxyflurane, meperidine, phenylbutazone, pyridoxyl phosphate-dependent enzymes, and theophylline; hence these drugs can lose their effects. Additive or superadditive effects can be expected when Seconal is combined with other CNS depressants such as narcotic analgesics, antihistamines, or tranquilizers. In a patient taking a heart drug such as the beta-blocker Inderal, beginning or stopping the use of a barbiturate may necessitate changing the dose of the heart drug.

See also BARBITURATES

Simethicone

Other name: polydimethylsiloxane
Source: synthesis
Pharmacology: antifoaming agent (surfactant)
Dose: This substance is not considered to be effective.

There are at least 17 products on the market (for example, Di-Gel, Gas-X, Gelusil, Mylanta) that ballyhoo simethicone as a defoaming agent that somehow will relieve pockets of gas that accumulate in the GI tract and that supposedly cause abdominal distress. However, an FDA advisory panel concluded that simethicone lacks evidence of effectiveness in treating abdominal discomfort associated with complaints of gas.

Gas in the GI tract is normal and healthy. Gas helps promote peristalsis and normal evacuation. Sometimes following surgery an "adynamic ileum" condition can arise in which a stagnant pocket of gas causes great distress, but this is far removed from normal gas production in everyday life. Certain foods seem to produce more gas in some people; these foods can be avoided if the gas becomes embarrassing or otherwise a problem.

In their decision the FDA also concluded that medical evidence indicates that there is no relationship between abdominal symptoms and the quantity of gas in the GI tract. It would appear that some drug companies and their advertising agencies are making a financial mountain out of a physiological molehill.

Misuse potential: high

Adverse effects: Simethicone is inert in the GI tract; it is not absorbed but is excreted unchanged.

See also ANTACIDS

Sinarest. *See* SINUS PRODUCTS

Sine-Aid. *See* SINUS PRODUCTS

Sine-Off. *See* SINUS PRODUCTS

Sinsemilla. *See* MARIJUANA

Sinus Products

The hollow cavities in the skull connecting with the nasal cavities are termed *sinuses.* One manifestation of the common cold is sinusitis—that is, infection and inflammation of any or all parts of the frontal, ethmoid, or maxillary sinuses. In full-blown sinusitis, the mucous membranes are swollen, the cavities cut off from breathing, and there can be pain or a burning sensation.

There is no drug you can take to cure the common cold or even hasten your recovery. But there are many products on the market that promise to relieve symptoms, including the symptoms of sinusitis.

These sinus products are remarkably alike in what they contain. First, they are all "shotgun" formulations, usually containing 3 different types of active ingredients. Second, they all contain a sympathomimetic that acts to shrink blood vessels in the swollen mucous membranes and thus somewhat open air passageways. These are called nasal decongestants. They come in tablet or nose drop form. The following table summarizes some of the popular sinus products:

| Trade Name | Ingredients Contained | | | | |
	Acetaminophen	Chlorpheniramine	Pseudoephedrine	Phenylpropanolamine	Other
Sinarest	yes	yes	—	yes	—
Sine-aid	yes	—	yes	—	—
Sine-off	—	yes	—	yes	aspirin
Sinutab	yes	yes	yes	—	—
Thrifty	yes	yes	yes	—	—
Tylenol Sinus	yes	—	yes	—	—

Acetaminophen and aspirin are painkillers. If there is no pain accompanying your sinus condition you don't need these ingredients or their possible adverse effects. Chlorpheniramine is an antihistamine. It cannot speed up your recovery, but it can make you sleepy and at risk if you drive a car. Pseudoephedrine and phenylpropanolamine (PPA) are sympathomimetics with vasoconstrictor action. They can temporarily relieve nasal stuffiness, but they can have adverse effects, too, especially in sensitive people. (These include insomnia, a too-fast heart rate, and possible high blood pressure.) Read the discussion of rebound effect and drug interactions using PPA in the section on PPA.

Left alone, the inflamed sinuses eventually will open up, drain, and return to normal. Decongestants can give only temporary relief; they can't speed recovery. And there always is the danger of overreliance on the decongestant. If the heavy, persuasive advertising convinces you that you need to use a sinus product, remember: All the ingredients in these shotgun products can be purchased singly as generic drugs at considerable savings.

See also ACETAMINOPHEN, ANTIHISTAMINES, ASPIRIN, COLD PRODUCTS, PHENYLPROPANOLAMINE, PSEUDOEPHEDRINE

Sinutab. *See* SINUS PRODUCTS

666 Cold Preparation

Other names of active ingredients: sodium salicylate, phenylpropanolamine
Source: compounding
Pharmacology: pain and fever reliever, decongestant
Dose: 1 caplet
Sold as a treatment for cold and cough, this misdesigned product epitomizes the true "shotgun" preparation. It contains sodium salicylate, phenylpropanolamine, ammonium chloride, sodium citrate, and magnesium sulfate. The FDA has come down hard on this product, stating that it lacks evidence of safety and effectiveness. For example, the sodium citrate and the ammonium chloride have no value in the treatment of the common cold or accompanying cough. There is nothing in this product that will cure a head cold.

Sodium salicylate and aspirin are chemically related, as both are derivatives of salicylic acid. If you are seeking pain or fever relief, generic aspirin is much cheaper than this product, and if you are allergic to aspirin, generic acetaminophen is a possible alternative. Phenylpropanolamine is discussed in its own section.

Misuse potential: high. There is no cure for the common cold, nor any drug that will speed up your recovery. The problem with shotgun products such as this is that a person must subject himself or herself to the possible adverse effects of 5 different drugs to obtain the possible benefits of any one drug.

Adverse effects: Some people are highly allergic to salicylates; they must avoid this product. Salicylates are known to "thin" the blood—that is, they prolong clotting time; they must not be used after any oral or general surgery where healing of a wound is occurring. Phenylpropanolamine is designed to have minimal effects upon the brain and heart, but in sensitive persons it can cause a too-rapid heartbeat and sleeplessness. If you have a history of heart problems, hyperthyroidism, glaucoma, or difficulty in emptying the bladder, avoid products that contain phenylpropanolamine.

Drug interactions: Taken together with other stimulants such as epinephrine, phenylpropanolamine can cause excessive stimulation of the heart, leading to rapid pulse and high blood pressure. Phenylpropanolamine works against the action of antihypertensive drugs. Irregular heartbeat can occur if phenylpropanolamine and digitalis are combined. The concurrent use of any monoamine oxidase inhibitor drug such as Parnate or Nardil is very dangerous because of the possibility of a very high rise in blood pressure (hypertensive crisis).

See also SALICYLATES, PHENYLPROPANOLAMINE

Sleep Aids

Insomnia, real or imagined, is a common occurrence in our population. Real insomnia may have its origin in thyroid disease, old age, disorders of the bladder or circulatory system, or in tension or neurosis. Imagined insomnia may result from overestimating the number of hours of sleep we need. Not everyone needs 8 hours of sleep a night; some can function well on 5. Furthermore, almost everyone occasionally experiences sleepless nights caused by the previous day's excitement, by a stuffy nose, or perhaps by a caffeine-containing drink. Some advertisers would have us believe that this is sufficient reason to rush out and buy a chemical crutch to get us through the night.

On the other hand, no one denies that to some people insomnia is a real, distressing, and recurrent problem. Often it is associated with psychological problems such as anxiety or depression. Getting at the cause of the insomnia is the best treatment, but that may entail a year's visits to a psychiatrist. The temptation is to turn to drugs, especially if they can be purchased without a prescription.

Among prescription drugs, the barbiturates have had the largest use as hypnotics (sleep-inducers). They are discussed in their own section. The benzodiazepines such as Librium and Valium were hailed as the safe substitutes for the barbiturates for sleep induction, but now we know that overreliance on them can easily lead to psychological and physical dependence (yet they are safer than the barbiturates). They, too, are discussed separately, as is Noludar.

Many insomniacs today rely on OTC products. The main ingredient in most OTC sleep aids is an antihistamine. Years ago it was discovered that one side effect of antihistamines is drowsiness; this effect has become the rationale for their use as sleep aids. The CNS depressant effect of the antihistamines that may help promote sleep also makes it dangerous to operate a car or machinery after taking these drugs. This is especially true if one combines alcohol with an antihistamine.

For many years, the antihistamine widely used in OTC sleep aids was methapyrilene. However, it was discovered that methapyrilene is a potent carcinogen in laboratory animals, and manufacturers quickly and quietly replaced it with either one of two other antihistamines—diphenhydramine or doxylamine. When manufacturers change active ingredients, they do not necessarily change the brand name; no regulation requires them to do so.

A survey of sleep aids on the market reveals the sameness of many of them. Many use the same active ingredient. For example, the antihistamine diphenhydramine is used in all of the following: Compoz (50 mg dose), Miles Nighttime Sleep Aid (25 mg), Nytol (25 mg), Sleep-Eze (25 mg), and Sominex (25 mg). The antihistamine doxylamine is found in all of the following: Contac (7.5 mg dose), NyQuil (7.5 mg), and Unisom (25 mg). For many of these products, then, your choice is not among drugs but among doses, prices, or attractive packaging. NOTE: One can purchase generic antihistamine OTC at a fraction of the cost of these very highly advertised brands.

Another ingredient in OTC sleep aids is scopolamine, an anticholinergic alkaloid obtained (along with atropine) from belladonna and henbane plants. In sufficient doses, scopolamine can cause drowsiness, amnesia, and dreamless sleep. Unpredictably, it may also induce excitement or hallucinations. Scopolamine has been used in obstetrics to cause a twilight sleep, a kind of amnesia in which the pain of delivery is felt but not remembered.

The important question is: Do the OTC sleep aids work? Users say emphatically, "Yes." Critics in the FDA and consumer advocate groups say, "At the doses recommended on the label, no." A dose of 25 mg of antihistamines or 0.5 mg of scopolamine is ineffective in sleep induction, they claim. For support, the critics cite a number of studies done in the past decade that cast much doubt on the advertising claims made for the OTC sleep aids. Other critics suggest that it is actually a placebo effect that helps the insomniac.

However, with the wide variations in human need and in the response to drugs, some insomniacs may be benefiting from these patent medicines. Others may be wasting their money. And for those who have become habituated to sleep aids and who must take them for the rest of their lives, the drugs may be worse than nothing at all.

Misuse potential: medium

Adverse effects: Your biggest concern in the use of sleep aids is the drowsiness you can experience the morning after you have taken them to get to sleep. Small amounts of the sleep aid will remain in your blood for more than 24 hours, and while this will not put you to sleep, it can make you less than alert mentally. This applies especially to the antihistamines and tranquilizers. And the more sleep aid you took, the longer and more intense will be the drowsiness you experience. Antihistamines should be used with caution in persons who have glaucoma, enlarged prostate, or difficulty urinating.

Drug interactions: All the sleep aids discussed here are brain depressants; if you combine them with any other depressant, including alcohol, you risk becoming so oversedated that you will not be able to function. Barbiturates are respiratory depressants as well, and their combination with alcohol (another respiratory depressant) can be fatal.

See also BARBITURATES, BENZODIAZEPINES, DOXYLAMINE, NOLUDAR, SCOPOLAMINE, VALIUM

Sloan's Liniment

Other name of active ingredient: methyl salicylate (oil of wintergreen)

Source: compounding

Pharmacology: counterirritant

Dose: applied externally

Promoted as an external painkiller, this misdesigned product is one of the best examples of the true "shotgun" preparation— that is, one that has a large number of ingredients in the hope that one of them will do some good. The FDA has firmly rejected Sloan's Liniment, concluding that it lacks evidence of safety or effectiveness.

Sloan's Liniment contains turpentine, kerosene, pine oil, camphor, methyl salicyclate, and capsicum oleoresin. Instead of subjecting yourself to all these expensive substances (and their possible adverse effects), treat pain with moist heat or generic aspirin, acetaminophen, or ibuprofen.

Misuse potential: high. You are unlikely to obtain significant, prolonged relief from this type of preparation. Furthermore, you are exposing yourself to six different substances, including kerosene and turpentine. There is no scientific evidence that these substances are safe and effective in a product to be used as a painkiller.

Adverse effects: Methyl salicylate is closely related to aspirin; if you have an aspirin or salicylate allergy, avoid this product. There have been reports of persons rubbing this type of liniment over very large areas of their body, with consequent absorption of very large quantities of methyl salicylate into their bloodstream. This can produce salicylate poisoning, especially in children. The poisoning is characterized by mental excitation, fever, rapid breathing, headache, ringing in the ears, dizziness, mental confusion, nausea, vomiting, and diarrhea. Accidental poisonings from oil of turpentine have occurred when too much of it has gotten into the system. The development of a skin rash indicates that you are sensitive to one or more of the ingredients in this product, most likely the methyl salicylate. If a rash develops, stop using this product immediately.

Drug interactions: Salicylates, including oil of wintergreen, may enhance the action of oral antidiabetic drugs (particularly Diabinese, one of the longer-acting hypoglycemics). This could result in a too-low blood sugar level and would require an adjustment in the dose of the oral hypoglycemic. A person taking the diuretic Lasix who also absorbs large doses of a salicylate has an increased risk of salicylate poisoning.

See also COUNTERIRRITANTS

Solvents and Inhalants

Other names: aerosol propellants, benzene, carbon tetrachloride, cleaning fluid, finger nail polish, gasoline, glue, paint thinner, rubber cement, spot remover, varnish

Source: petroleum, synthesis

Pharmacology: brain depressants, deliriants

Dose: variable; by inhalation

Most of the sniffing of solvents and inhalants is done by teenagers (or younger) who seem to want to put themselves into a delirious, semiconscious state of altered awareness. They call this getting high. One sniffer said that when he inhaled gasoline, he felt like he was floating through the air. Actually, these persons are replacing the oxygen in their inhaled breath with a hydrocarbon or other solvent that can have a brain-depressant action or a heart-stimulant action. As more of the substance is inhaled, the person can become restless, excited, confused, disoriented, or finally comatose. When these chemicals are inhaled there is a real danger of dying of asphyxiation.

Hydrocarbons of the gasoline, benzene, paint thinner, and varnish type can depress the brain but also can sensitize the heart to the point where fibrillation and sudden death can occur. With smaller doses, eye irritation, headache, nausea, dizziness, and weakness can be expected. Glue sniffing in children can cause exhilaration, euphoria, excitement, slurred speech, and double vision. Stupor and unconsciousness may follow.

Propellants in common use today are of the fluorochlorohydrocarbon type (similar to the Freons). Sniffing of such aerosol sprays can be extremely hazardous because the heart can be sensitized to the point where fibrillation occurs. This is more likely to happen with high doses of aerosol sniffed in confined spaces.

Abuse potential: high

Adverse effects: No matter what solvent or chemical is inhaled, asphyxiation is an ever-present hazard. All of the solvents (with the exception of carbon tetrachloride and certain aerosols) are highly flammable; a lighted cigarette could easily ignite them. Carbon tetrachloride and benzene are known to cause cancer in laboratory animals, and presumably also in humans. The vasodilator effects of the volatile nitrites are discussed in the section on nitrites.

Drug interactions: Most of the solvents and inhalants discussed here depress the brain, and the use of any other depressant such as alcohol will add to that depression. The use of epinephrine, amphetamines, or caffeine during the exposure to gasoline or the aerosol propellants can increase the chance of ventricular fibrillation.

See also NITRITES, NITROUS OXIDE

Soma. *See* MEPROBAMATE

Spanish Fly

Main ingredient: cantharidin
Source: insects
Pharmacology: blistering agent (vesicant)
Dose: no rational use in medicine

The much-discussed, supposed aphrodisiac Spanish fly consists of dried insects of the genus *Cantharis,* from Spain or Russia. The insects contain cantharidin, a lactone that acts as an irritant stimulant to the reproductive and urinary organs.

When Spanish fly is ingested, the genitals can become swollen and painful, with possible membrane rupture. Some individuals may interpret this condition as sexual stimulation, but emergency room personnel have long held a different opinion. They know that cantharidin is a powerful blistering agent and that swollen genitals and ruptured membranes hardly constitute sexual stimulation. Spanish fly is hardly an aphrodisiac.

Large brown capsules labeled "Spanish fly" are sold on the street with no indication of source, dosage, or precautions. One has no idea what one is ingesting in such a situation. Spanish fly also is known as Russian fly, blistering beetle, and cantharides.

Abuse potential: high

Adverse effects: Taken orally, this preparation can cause vomiting, abdominal pain, and shock. When it reaches the urinary bladder, it causes a constant urge to urinate. In the urethra it causes the penis to swell, but the possibility of kidney damage makes it a dangerous drug to use. The active ingredient, cantharidin, is intensely irritating to mucous membranes.

See also APHRODISIACS

Speed. *See* AMPHETAMINES, METHAMPHETAMINE

Sports, Drugs in. *See* DRUGS IN SPORTS

Stanozolol. *See* ANABOLIC STEROIDS, STEROIDS

Steroids

Steroids are found in the plant and animal kingdoms and also are made synthetically. They are large molecules made of carbon, hydrogen, and oxygen atoms. Steroids all have a fused, 17-carbon ring structure, with many variations that confer special drug properties. Steroids usually are very potent drugs, effective in milligram doses. They must not be used casually, nor should your prescription be shared with friends.

The most abused steroid drugs today are the anabolic steroids (see that section), used by certain athletes in the expectation of building body mass. Estrogen, a steroidal female sex hormone, is widely used by menopausal women and often is misused by women who take it for too long a time, or who take it in the hope of postponing the effects of old age. (See the section on estrogen.)

Most steroids are available by prescription only and are neither abused nor misused. The following table summarizes steroidal categories and examples; both naturally occurring and synthetic steroids are represented.

See also ANABOLIC STEROIDS, ESTROGENS

Stimulant Drugs. *See* AMPHETAMINES, CAFFEINE, COCAINE, NICOTINE, RITALIN, SYMPATHOMIMETICS

STP. *See* HALLUCINOGENIC AMPHETAMINE DERIVATIVES

Sudafed. *See* PSEUDOEPHEDRINE

Steroid Category	Examples	Comments
anabolic	Deca-Durabolin, Kabolin, Nadrolone, Oxandrolone, Oxymetholone, Stanozolol	Prescribed for debilitated patients; wide use in sports to gain competitive edge.
anti-inflammatory	Dexamethasone, Prednisone, Triamcinolone	Also used as anti-itching agents; affect electrolyte balance, carbohydrate metabolism; inflammatory response.
bile salts	sodium glycocholate	Help emulsify fat in the intestine.
birth control pills	ethynodiol, norethindrone	Mimic the effects of progesterone; inhibit ovulation.
hormone of pregnancy	progesterone	Prepares and maintains the uterus in pregnancy.
mineralocorticosteroids	aldosterone	Affect electrolyte balance.
lipids	cholesterol	Found throughout the body; significant factor in hardening of the arteries.
plant steroids	digitalis	Potent heart stimulant (cardiotonic).
sex hormones	estradiol, testosterone	Establish secondary sex characteristics.
vitamin D precursor	ergosterol	Upon irradiation with sunlight or UV light is converted to active vitamin D.

Sympathomimetics

To be classified as a sympathomimetic, a drug must produce actions that mimic or resemble the physiologic response we observe when the sympathetic division of the autonomic nervous system is stimulated. Sympathetic nerve discharge controls the "fight or flight" response and results in increased blood pressure, dilation of bronchi and pupil of the eye, stimulation of the brain, constriction of blood vessels in the skin, increased blood glucose levels, and diminished peristalsis and digestive juice flow. Hence a sympathetic drug could be expected to produce most or all of these body responses.

The catecholamines (epinephrine, norepinephrine, dopamine) are the body's own, natural sympathomimetics. We release them in response to stress, fright, or anger, and they produce all of the fight or flight responses listed in the preceding paragraph. Ephedrine is a sympathomimetic from a plant.

Many synthetic sympathomimetics are available. The amphetamines are used in medicine for their ability to excite the CNS (as in narcolepsy, minimal brain dysfunction) and to depress appetite in weight control programs. Betaphenethylamine analogs (Neo-Synephrine, Isuprel inhaler, Sudafed, Wyamine, phenylpropanolamine, pseudoephedrine, Paredrine, Vasoxyl, Orthoxine, Privine, Visine) are used variously as sinus and nasal decongestants, vasoconstrictors (in eye drops), agents to raise blood pressure, and as bronchodilators in asthma. Phenylpropanolamine and pseudoephedrine (discussed in their own sections) are found in dozens of products. What the consumer must remember is that when an OTC sympathomimetic is used to depress the appetite, shrink nasal membranes, or treat asthma, serious adverse effects may be experienced. All the sympathomimetics have some ability to excite the brain and heart or to raise blood pressure. In most people this is of little consequence, but in children, heart patients, insomniacs, or other sensitive users, the adverse effects become important enough to warrant discontinuance or avoidance of the drug. For example, some users of Sudafed can experience restlessness, insomnia, and dryness of the mouth and throat. The same effects can be experienced by persons using Acutrim, Dexatrim, Prolamine, or other appetite-suppressant products. An asthmatic using an epinephrine inhaler might discover that his or her appetite is affected by the stimulant drug. All these adverse effects are much more pronounced if the drug has been taken orally; the same drug in nose drop or eye drop form is less likely to produce adverse effects.

Drug interactions: Remember also that when you use a sympathomimetic as an OTC or prescription drug, you are exposing yourself to the risk of drug interactions. The most dangerous of these is the interaction with monoamine oxidase inhibitors such as Parnate or Nardil, which can produce dangerously high blood pressure and brain excitation. Be sure to avoid this combination of drugs; your pharmacist can tell you which drugs to avoid. Sympathomimetics can interfere with the antihypertensive effects of methyldopa and reserpine.

See also AMPHETAMINES, COLD REMEDIES

T

Talacen. *See* TALWIN

Talwin

Other names: pentazocine, Talacen
Source: synthesis
Pharmacology: analgesic painkiller
Dose: By injection, 30 mg every 3–4 hours; total daily dose should not exceed 360 mg. Orally, 1 50-mg tablet every 3–4 hours; total daily dosage should not exceed 12 tablets. NOTE: Talwin tablets, intended strictly for oral use, are formulated with 0.5 mg of the narcotic antagonist naloxone. When taken by mouth, the naloxone does not interfere with the action of the Talwin, but if a drug user attempts to dissolve the tablets and inject the solution, the naloxone blocks the action of the Talwin. This approach is designed to discourage street abuse of Talwin tablets.

This analgesic is intended for the relief of moderate to severe pain. It has been used extensively in surgery as a pre- and postoperative medication and is about a third as powerful as morphine in relieving pain. Because it works on the same brain receptors as the opiates, it is considered by law a narcotic and therefore is a controlled substance under the 1970 Controlled Substances Act. Illegal possession or possession with the intent to sell is a federal crime.

Talwin was one of the first mixed agonist/antagonist opioids—that is, it demonstrated both narcotic and antinarcotic properties. It is a narcotic because it attaches to brain receptors, producing pain relief. It is a narcotic antagonist because it blocks (albeit weakly) the effects of morphine and partially reverses breathing depression caused by that drug. The explanation for this dual, apparently contradictory action lies in the compound's special chemical structure, which controls its binding to the receptor. Talwin binds and has a pharmacologic action of its own, but its presence on the receptor keeps other drugs such as morphine from binding and working.

Talacen is a fixed-dose combination of pentazocine with acetaminophen (650 mg); this combination of drugs works better than either drug alone to relieve pain and fever.

Abuse potential: high. Unfortunately, pentazocine has become a drug of abuse among physicians and others. It comes as a solution for injection and can be mainlined very easily. On the street it sometimes is mixed with pyribenzamine as a cheap substitute for heroin. Physical dependence on Talwin can develop, and a withdrawal syndrome has been observed. Therefore, use of Talwin in large doses or for greater than 4–5 days involves some risk, especially if it is injected. WARNING: Patients with a history of drug use, or emotionally unstable persons, are at greater risk of abusing pentazocine; close observation of such patients is indicated.

Adverse effects: Adverse reactions to Talwin include nausea, vomiting, dizziness, hallucinations, confusion, disorientation, sweating, and infrequently nightmares.

Drug interactions: Drug interactions with pentazocine appear to be rare. It may have the potential for causing a rise in a body enzyme called serum amylase; since serum amylase levels are used by physicians to diagnose diseases, this could cause a diagnostic problem.

CAUTION: Do not substitute Talwin for other narcotics as it may precipitate an acute withdrawal reaction.

See NARCOTIC ANALGESICS

Tanning Pills

Although it is illegal openly to sell tanning pills in the United States, they still are available by mail order. These pills contain beta-carotene, a yellow-to-yellow-red pigment found in carrots, sweet potatoes, milk fat, leafy vegetables, and egg yolks. These sources usually also contain canthaxanthin, another highly colored pigment.

When large amounts of beta-carotene are ingested, the yellowish pigment accumulates in the palms, soles of the feet, stool, blood, and after about a week in the skin, where it gives the appearance of a tan. Health faddists who drink very large quantities of carrot juice sometimes find that their palms and soles have turned yellow.

Beta-carotene alone is not toxic in the human, but ingesting large quantities of it along with canthaxanthin may result in damage to the retina of the eye as well as the depositing of fat in the liver, blood, and skin. For this reason tanning pills are to be avoided.

Carotene exists in various forms, designated alpha, beta, and gamma. These forms are provitamin A compounds convertible to vitamin A in the body. A deficiency of vitamin A in the human is associated with night blindness and damage to the white of the eye and the cornea.

Teratogens

The use or abuse of certain drugs during pregnancy can have disastrous consequences on the unborn child. A substance capable of causing birth defects in the developing embryo or fetus is termed a teratogen. The first trimester of pregnancy is the most critical. The actual defect may be physical: malformed limbs, face, heart, or other organ or joint. Or it may be mental: brain damage, mental retardation. The damage may be subtle or overwhelming. Besides chemical agents (drugs, environmental poisons), X rays, gamma rays, and other forms of radiation can act teratogenically.

Thalidomide is the most infamous teratogen; alcohol is the most common. Since the estrogen in birth control pills can act teratogenically, it is very important that birth control pills *not* be taken for even a day if pregnancy is suspected. The list of possible teratogens is so great that the pregnant woman is well advised to expose her fetus to no drug, no chemical, no alcohol, and no radiation unless her physician approves.

The FDA has established 5 pregnancy categories to indicate a drug's teratogenic potential. For drugs that might be given during pregnancy, the label must indicate to which category the drug belongs. The categories are:

- Category A: Studies indicate no teratogenicity; risk to fetus is remote.
- Category B: Either animal studies are negative but there have been no studies in women, or animal studies are positive but studies in women are negative for teratogenicity. Hence risk to the fetus is low.
- Category C: Either animal studies are positive for teratogenicity but studies in women have not been reported, or there is no information from either animal or human studies. Decision to use or not is based on risk/benefit considerations.
- Category D: Enough evidence has been gathered from human studies to indicate a clear risk of teratogenicity in pregnant women. Drug is contraindicated in all but the most serious or life-threatening situations.
- Category X: There is little or no doubt that the drug is a teratogen, based upon animal and/or human studies. Drug should not be used by pregnant women.

For years consumer groups have been conducting an anticaffeine campaign, aimed most recently at pregnant women. From data on animals and humans, the groups believe that caffeine is linked to such birth defects as cleft palate, heart abnormalities, and missing fingers and toes. Letters have been sent to thousands of obstetricians, gynecologists, and midwives, urging them to advise women to avoid caffeine (coffee, tea, colas, OTC products) during pregnancy. The FDA, however, has said that their tests have failed to demonstrate any conclusive evidence against caffeine as a cause of birth defects. Just the same, the FDA wants caffeine-containing products to be labeled to warn pregnant women and nursing mothers to avoid their use.

Phocomelia is the array of rare birth defects in the form of seal-like flippers in place of arms or legs, or sometimes the complete absence of limbs. These worst-case teratogenic effects were seen with Thalidomide; some 8000 babies in 20 countries were afflicted.

Certain street drugs have long been criticized as causing birth defects. However, when one looks for scientific evidence to support the claims, one usually finds less than convincing data. For example, LSD often has been labeled a teratogen, but while some evidence has been found, scientific proof still is lacking. Three studies have implicated marijuana in birth defects, but polydrug use in the women studied made it difficult to pinpoint teratogenicity. One thing we do know: Among the dozens of street drugs and chemicals routinely abused, including especially the new designer drugs, the structural potential exists for causing serious birth defects. The only way a pregnant woman can be sure she is protected is to avoid all such drug use.

See also ALCOHOL, CAFFEINE

Testing for Drugs. *See* DRUGS, TESTING FOR

THC (tetrahydrocannabinol). *See* MARIJUANA

Tigan

Other name: trimethobenzamide
Source: synthesis
Pharmacology: antiemetic (control of vomiting)
Dose: individualized. Adults, usually 250 mg 3–4 times a day. Children, 30–90 pounds, 1–2 100-mg capsules 3–4 times a day. Or 1 suppository for adults 3–4 times a day; children, 30–90 pounds, ½ to 1 suppository 3–4 times a day.

The manufacturers describe Tigan as an antiemetic agent for the control of nausea and vomiting in adults and children. However, they are quick to point out that Tigan is not indicated for simple vomiting in children, but rather for extended vomiting whose cause is known. The reason for this caution is clear: There appears to be a link between the use of centrally acting antiemetics in the control of virus-caused vomiting, and the very serious acute condition called Reye syndrome (see the section on Reye syndrome). The evidence for the link is tenuous but does suggest that drugs like Tigan be used with caution.

Further, Tigan can damage the liver, and this makes the symptoms of Reye syndrome even worse.

All this suggests that the physician and the parent take steps to avoid the use of Tigan or any antiemetic in children who have chicken pox, measles, or any illness that acts like the flu.

Adverse effects: Tigan can cause headache, blurred vision, low blood pressure, drowsiness, or skin rash.

Drug interactions: Combining Tigan with any other CNS-depressant drug such as alcohol, antihistamines, tranquilizers, or sedatives can result in oversedation.

TMA. *See* HALLUCINOGENIC AMPHETAMINE DERIVATIVES

Tobacco. *See* NICOTINE

Tolerance

In drug abuse or misuse, tolerance can be a major factor in how seriously one gets hurt by the drug.

Tolerance to a drug is the development of a condition in which ever larger and larger doses of the drug must be taken to obtain the desired result. In other words, the drug doesn't seem to work anymore, and you have to take more of it.

Tolerance can develop to alcohol, nicotine, Valium, barbiturates, heroin, morphine (and to all the opiates and opioids), LSD, and to many other drugs. In one verified case a morphine addict had worked his way up to 5000 mg of it daily; he had developed a prodigious tolerance. Some smokers go through 3 packs of cigarettes a day; they are highly tolerant to nicotine. However, tolerance may develop to some effects of a drug but not to others. With alcohol and barbiturates, tolerance may occur with respect to the dose required to impair performance on certain tasks, but the lethal dose of alcohol or barbiturates is not that different for tolerant versus nontolerant people.

How quickly one may develop tolerance depends on the frequency and size of the dose and the route of administration. Large, frequent, intravenous doses of a drug all predispose to the development of tolerance. You may have no choice in the matter, but if you do, try to cut down on the size of the dose and take the drug by mouth. In this way there is not such a heavy burden put on the liver to detoxify it.

Barbiturates offer the classical example. An occasional dose to get to sleep may progress to nightly use. When the original dose fails to produce sleep, it is increased. A month or so later it may be up to 2–3 times the original dose. Six months later the tolerance is extraordinary and the person may be taking hundreds of milligrams to get to sleep. Hand in hand with the tolerance, the person likely has developed a physical dependency on the barbiturates. He or she is hooked.

The development of tolerance can be understood by considering the enzymes in the liver that the body uses in the normal biotransformation of drugs. Repeated, large doses of a drug can stimulate (induce) the liver to make a larger supply of these enzymes. So the person takes a larger dose to compensate, but this only induces the synthesis of more enzyme. Hence a vicious cycle is established; the person has developed tolerance. He or she has only two alternatives: Take ever-increasing doses of the drug, or stop it altogether.

See also ADDICTION, BARBITURATES, NARCOTIC ANALGESICS

Toxicity

The toxicity of a substance is the measure of its poisonous character. Some substances, such as cyanide or dioxin, are highly poisonous, causing death or damage in milligram amounts. Other substances are toxic only if grams of them are ingested. We can quantify toxicity by the use of the LD_{50}, the quantity of material that, when ingested or applied to the skin in a single dose, will kill 50% of the test animals (usually rodents). The LD_{50} is expressed in grams or milligrams per kilogram of animal body weight so that data are comparable.

The *lower* the LD_{50} value, the more toxic the substance. The LD_{50} of dioxin is only 22 mcg/kg in the male rat, making dioxin one of the most poisonous chemicals known. The LD_{50} of paraquat is 57 mg/kg orally in the rat; that of chloroform is 3.28 g/kg in the mouse, subcutaneously. Another term, the LC_{50}, measures the concentration in air that causes the death of 50% of the test animals.

Toxicity can be acute or chronic. Acute toxicity is damage to the body as the result of single or short-duration exposure. For example, a youth smoking his or her first cigarette may suffer from acute nicotine poisoning, or a worker may be hospitalized after exposure to chlorine fumes. Chronic toxicity is damage as the result of repeated or long-term exposure to lesser quantities of the toxin. Examples are liver cirrhosis from years of alcohol abuse, or the cumulative effects of lead poisoning over a period of time. Actually, toxicity may not manifest itself until years after the original exposure to the poison (this is called the latent period). Examples are cancer of the lung from asbestos exposure or cigarette smoke, and cataracts of the eye from radiation.

Before a new drug is marketed, the manufacturer carries out tests for acute and chronic toxicity, carcinogenicity (causing malignancies), teratogenicity (producing malformed fetuses), and mutagenicity (causing heritable changes). No drug or chemical is ever completely free of some degree of toxicity, even though it might be slight or affect only a small percentage of those exposed to it. Even oxygen, essential to life, can cause eye damage to a newborn infant if the exposure is too great. It is important to keep in mind that the drugs on the market are typically foreign to our body, have the potential for serious side effects, and it would be better if possible to avoid use of the drug in favor of some nondrug treatment.

Through the Environmental Protection Agency (EPA) and the Occupational Safety and Health Act (OSHA), our government monitors conditions in the workplace and in the environment generally. OSHA has identified dozens of hazardous chemicals and has set permissible exposure limits (PELs) for the workplace. Threshold limit values (TLVs) are published for a large number of chemicals. A TLV is a condition or concentration of a substance under which it is believed that nearly all workers may be repeatedly exposed day after day without adverse effects.

The concentrations of toxic air and water pollutants are measured in parts per million (PPM), parts per billion (PPB), or milligrams per cubic meter (mg/mm^3).

See also CARCINOGEN, TERATOGEN

Tranquilizers, Minor

Other names: antianxiety agents, anxiolytics, benzodiaze-
pines, carbamates
Source: synthesis
Pharmacology: short-term relief of anxiety, insomnia; skele-
tal muscle relaxants
Dose: typically, 5–25 mg

When most people refer to "tranquilizers" they mean the
minor tranquilizers, those drugs used to treat anxiety neuroses.
(Major tranquilizers are used to treat psychotic states such as
schizophrenia.) Minor tranquilizers are useful in calming anxious persons, neurotics fearful of life's situations, or those so
tense that they cannot function or sleep normally. The minor
tranquilizers are of little or no benefit in the treatment of schizophrenia or other psychoses; rather, they are prescribed for
people who still are in touch with reality.

Neurotic persons have not lost touch with reality but can
suffer acutely from anxiety ("I know I have cancer," or "I know
I will never get a job") or from phobia (germs, heights, closed-in
places, other people). To the neurotic, these feelings can be
very real; and when they are accompanied by palpitation of the
heart, choking sensations, dizziness, or breathlessness, treatment is necessary. The true insomniac also has a very real problem, one that has in the past been treated too often with barbiturates. The minor tranquilizers offer a much safer alternative
to sleep induction. As shown in the following table, minor tranquilizers fall into one of two chemical classifications: the benzodiazepines or the propanediol carbamates.

The minor tranquilizers of the benzodiazepine type are exemplified by Valium. They were introduced in the 1960s as
effective CNS depressants for treating anxiety, muscle spasm,
and sleep disorders. They were the physician's answer to the
dangerous barbiturates and were an instant therapeutic success, heavily prescribed by doctors and eagerly sought by patients. The benzodiazepine tranquilizers appeared safe because
it was virtually impossible to commit suicide with them. In
1977, 90 million prescriptions were written for minor tranquilizers. Today, in any given year, about 11% of all Americans will
take a minor tranquilizer.

Generic Name	Trade Name	Half-life (hours)	Typical Oral Adult Dose (mg)
Benzodiazepine type			
alprazolam	Xanax	4–20	0.25–4.0 daily*
chlorazepate	Tranxene	24–72	15–60 daily*
chlordiazepoxide	Librium	24–72	5–25 3–4 times daily
clonazepam	Clonopin	24–72	1.5–20 daily*
diazepam	Valium	24–72	2–10 2–4 times daily
flurazepam	Dalmane	24–72	15–30 at bedtime
halazepam	Paxipam	24–72	20–40 3 or 4 times daily
lorazepam	Ativan	4–20	2–6 daily*
oxazepam	Serax	4–20	10–15 3–4 times daily
prazepam	Centrax	24–72	20–60 daily*
temazepam	Restoril	4–20	15–30 before retiring
triazolam	Halcion	4–20	0.25–0.50 before retiring
Propanediol carbamate type			
meprobamate	Equanil, Miltown	10	400 3 times daily
carisoprodol	Soma, Rela	c. 10	350 4 times daily

*In divided doses

But as we have seen before, there can be a later unfortunate phase in the pattern of new drug introduction. The safety of the minor tranquilizers, combined with their usefulness and acceptance, disarmed physicians, who began to prescribe them casually and often without supervision. In too many patients, occasional use became months-long or year-long use, and the destructive potential of these drugs became evident. In particular, Valium seemed to be in everyone's medicine chest and pocketbook as well as on the street.

More than 15 years of use passed before society recognized that, while brief use of minor tranquilizers can be very beneficial, long-term use or heavy dosage can and does lead to physical addiction. Chronic users who abruptly stop these medications can undergo a withdrawal syndrome that may be worse than that from heroin—indeed, it may be life-threatening. It took that long to realize that there is little reason to use a minor tranquilizer for longer than a month and that to do so can increase the risk of dependence. By the 1980s self-help groups such as Pill Addicts Anonymous had been organized to help people deal with the very drugs they were relying on to cope with their original problems. It is now known that benzodiazepine addicts need as much support as alcoholics, especially since secondary withdrawal symptoms from benzodiazepines commonly last for 18 months to 2 years. (In secondary withdrawal, the same abstinence symptoms—nightmares, agitation, anxiety, tremors, cramps, diarrhea—that accompanied the original withdrawal can recur months or years later.)

Benzodiazepine tranquilizers continue to be very popular. Valium has dropped from its number 1 position as the nation's top newly prescribed drug, but it still is in the top 10. Dalmane is in the top 15; Ativan and Tranxene are in the top 30. In the past 20 years, tranquilizers have become intrinsic to our way of life.

Studies have shown that unexpectedly high rates of minor tranquilizer use occur among housewives, retired persons, and others who are unemployed. For example, while women who are unemployed or not in the labor force make up only 26% of the general population, they account for 46% of minor tranquilizer use. On the other hand, skilled and semiskilled workers have one of the lowest use rates.

What have we learned from the record of use of the minor

tranquilizers? Are drugs the answer to solving emotional problems? Is relief "just a pill away"? Perhaps the story of these drugs has taught us that "safe and effective" isn't necessarily good; that drugs can change cultural values; that there can be a potential for danger that is revealed only after years of drug use; that some tension and stress are normal, and that we should think twice about relying on a chemical crutch; that psychoactive drugs must never be prescribed casually and without supervision; and that the character needed to handle one's problems cannot be acquired by the use of any medication.

Abuse potential: high. Because the minor tranquilizers *appear* to be safe and because they are so available on prescription, people tend to overrely on them to handle stress or to get to sleep. Overreliance can lead to tolerance, greater doses, and ultimately dependence.

Adverse effects: The benzodiazepine and meprobamate types of minor tranquilizers are to be avoided during pregnancy because there is evidence that they can cause birth defects. This evidence is based on findings with only a few of the minor tranquilizers but appears to be applicable to all. If a patient is maintained on minor tranquilizers for longer than a month, blood and liver tests should be done to ensure that no damage to these organs is occurring. Other adverse effects to be expected in some users of minor tranquilizers are: drowsiness (ask your doctor if you can cut down on the dose to reduce this), dizziness, stomach upset, blurred vision, headache, skin rash, double vision, slurred speech, mental confusion, and changes in sex drive. Of course, not every patient will experience all these adverse effects. In a very few users, the minor tranquilizers produce totally unexpected effects, including anger, insomnia, depression, hyperexcitation, and nightmares. This is just another indication of biological variation; it shows how different many of us are.

Drug interactions: Oversedation can occur if a minor tranquilizer is combined with another brain depressant such as an antihistamine, a narcotic analgesic, or especially with alcohol. If a benzodiazepine type of minor tranquilizer is combined with a monoamine oxidase inhibitor drug such as Parnate or Nardil, oversedation may occur.

See also BENZODIAZEPINES, MEPROBAMATE, VALIUM

Tronolane. *See* PRAMOXINE

Tums. *See* ANTACIDS

Tylenol. *See* ACETAMINOPHEN

Tylenol-Sinus. *See* SINUS PRODUCTS

U

Urine Testing. *See* DRUGS, TESTING FOR

V

Valium

Other name: diazepam
Source: synthesis
Pharmacology: control of tension and anxiety; relief of muscle spasm; in alcohol withdrawal; for insomnia
Dose: individualized. For anxiety in adults, 2–10 mg 2–4 times a day. For skeletal muscle spasm, 2–10 mg 3–4 times a day. Geriatric patients require less. In children use smallest effective dose. Valium is supplied in tablets of 2 mg (white), 5 mg (yellow), and 10 mg (blue).

Introduced in 1964, Valium was hailed as the safe alternative to the barbiturates for the treatment of anxiety, muscle spasm, and insomnia. In severe stage of alcohol withdrawal, Valium may be useful in treating agitation, tremor, or impending delirium tremens. It appears to be useful in relief of skeletal muscle spasm caused by injury, inflammation, or nerve disorders.

Because it does not depress respiration significantly (when used in the absence of other drugs), it is virtually impossible to commit suicide with Valium. Acceptance by physicians and the public made Valium an instant success, and it has been in the top most-prescribed drugs in the United States for many years. Experts consider it a valuable drug.

In a 2- or 5-mg dose, diazepam will not depress REM sleep. However, a 5-mg dose can cause driving impairment equivalent to a 0.07% blood alcohol concentration. (If one's job demands mental alertness, Valium may be contraindicated.) The combination of Valium and alcohol is *much* more dangerous than Valium alone and is capable of causing death from respiratory depression. Valium is intended for use in neurotics but not in psychotics. It is now available generically on prescription at a lower cost.

The original secure, confident attitude about diazepam has given way to caution. We now know that tolerance and physical dependence on this drug can occur if it is taken for a long time. Withdrawal symptoms can occur after taking large doses (such as 100 mg a day) for a few days, moderate doses for a few months, and small doses (5–20 mg a day) for a few years. Severe withdrawal is characterized by anxiety, restlessness, tremors, nausea, cramps, diarrhea, muscle spasms, tics, moodiness, confusion, disorganized thinking, racing thoughts, bizarre dreams, hallucinations, paranoia, violence, depression, and possibly convulsions that can be life-threatening. Ironically, Valium addicts today can join a self-help group known as Pill Addicts Anonymous. The "safe" drug has itself become a threat to society.

Abuse potential: high. Because Valium is so heavily prescribed and because it appears to be so safe to use, it is easy to overrely on it for the treatment of stress and insomnia. Overreliance leads to tolerance, ever larger doses, and ultimately dependence. If you must use this drug at all, restrict your use to a few days and certainly not more than a week (unless your physician has so directed). Withdrawal from Valium dependence is potentially a life-threatening process because of the high likelihood of convulsions. Withdrawal should not be attempted alone; seek medical help.

Adverse effects: Valium and the other benzodiazepine-type minor tranquilizers are to be avoided during pregnancy because there is evidence that they can cause birth defects. This evidence is based upon findings with only a few of the minor tranquilizers, but appears to be applicable to all. If a patient is maintained on Valium for longer than a month, blood and liver tests should be done to check for possible damage. Valium users have reported the following adverse effects: drowsiness, fatigue, muscular incoordination, double vision, constipation, confusion, headache, depression, skin rash, stomach upset, slurred speech, and changes in sex drive. In a very few users, Valium causes totally unexpected effects, including anger, depression, insomnia, hyperexcitation, and nightmares. Usually there is no way to predict who will react in this bizarre way.

Drug interactions: You are strongly urged to avoid mixing alcohol and Valium (or any other tranquilizer). The combination is especially effective in depressing the brain. Other drugs that can potentiate the action of Valium include phenothiazines such as Thorazine, Haldol, and Mellaril, narcotic painkillers, barbiturates, and monoamine oxidase inhibitors such as Parnate and Nardil. Elimination of Valium from the body can be delayed if the drug is combined with Tagamet.

See also BENZODIAZEPINES, TRANQUILIZERS (MINOR)

Valmid

Other name: ethinamate
Source: synthesis
Pharmacology: short-acting hypnotic (sleep-inducer)
Dose: 0.5–1.0 g (1–2 capsules) 20 minutes before retiring. In the elderly, limit the dose to 1 capsule if possible.

As a treatment for insomnia, this drug has an unusually large dose, and its duration of action, about 4 hours, is relatively short. It is part of a group of CNS depressants that are loosely related chemically and that includes Doriden, Noludar, methaqualone, and Placidyl. They are not barbiturates, but their pharmacology is similar to that of barbiturates.

The manufacturer cautions against the use of Valmid for more than a few days, for tolerance can develop upon lengthy use, and there is the real possibility of the development of physical dependence. There are other hazards in the use of this hypnotic. Very large doses can cause death through respiratory depression. Recovering alcoholics who take it in support of their detoxification may find it quite euphoric and thus develop a psychic dependence on it.

Abuse potential: medium. The risk is the same as with many brain-depressant drugs: It is easy to overrely on them, to increase their dose as tolerance develops, and ultimately to become dependent on them. The dependence on Valmid can be physical: Abruptly stopping its use can result in a withdrawal syndrome. In the case of Valmid, the withdrawal can include life-threatening convulsions.

Adverse effects: If you take Valmid to get to sleep, the next morning you can still be groggy enough to make driving a car or operating machinery hazardous. The safety of Valmid in pregnancy has not been established; do not take this drug if you are pregnant or expect to become pregnant. If you are nursing a baby, do not take this drug without first consulting with your doctor. Some users of Valmid report skin rashes or stomach upset. Children who take this drug may unexpectedly become excited by it.

Drug interactions: CAUTION: Do not combine this drug with alcohol, as the combination can result in overdepression of the brain. The same applies to other depressants, including antihistamines, tranquilizers, and barbiturates. With these combinations you are at risk if you drive a car or engage in other activities that require mental alertness. Drugs of the Valmid type have been known to prevent oral anticoagulant drugs from working.

See also BARBITURATES

Vanquish

Other names of active ingredients: acetaminophen, aspirin
Source: compounding
Pharmacology: pain and fever reliever
Dose: 2 tablets (called "caplets"), each containing 194 mg of acetaminophen and 227 mg of aspirin

This product contains both aspirin and acetaminophen, an irrational combination because taken together these two analgesics are no more effective than taken singly, but by ingesting both of these drugs you risk the side effects of both. What is more, Vanquish contains caffeine—a stimulant that cannot relieve pain but can cause sleeplessness, heart arrhythmias, and tremors. The FDA has ruled that for treating headache caffeine is not a safe and effective drug. Caffeine will not relieve the symptoms of arthritis, sore muscle, or sore throat. There is no cure for the common cold, nor even a drug that will hasten recovery from it.

Vanquish, selling for about $3.49 for 60 tablets, is expensive. Similar, generic products sell for $2.59 for 100 tablets.

Misuse potential: medium

Adverse effects: Persons who are allergic to aspirin must avoid this product. Aspirin can "thin" the blood—that is, it prolongs bleeding time; for this reason aspirin products should not be used after or before surgery of any kind. (Note that the manufacturers recommend this product be used after "dental procedures.") Because there is evidence that use of aspirin in children may be associated with Reye syndrome, do not use this product for the relief of fever in children who have a viral infection without first consulting your physician. Caffeine is a brain stimulant and can cause wakefulness; in some sensitive persons it can cause heart arrhythmias. In recommended doses, acetaminophen probably will not produce significant adverse effects. But large doses of it can damage the liver.

Drug interactions: If you are taking an oral anticoagulant (that is, a drug that will prevent clotting) and you combine it with this product, your blood may be "thinned" so much that spontaneous hemorrhaging may occur. Aspirin can irritate the stomach; combining it with alcohol can increase the irritation. If you are taking a drug to lower blood sugar (such as Orinase or Diabinese) and you combine it with this product, you may experience too great a lowering of blood sugar. Aspirin will work against the antiarthritic actions of Anturane and Benemid. If you are taking any prescription medication, consult your physician before taking this product.

See also ASPIRIN, ACETAMINOPHEN

Vaporub. *See* COUNTERIRRITANTS

Varnish. *See* SOLVENTS AND INHALANTS

"Vitamin B-15"

The FDA believes that the various "vitamin B-15" products on the market today are hoaxes, frauds, and possibly dangerous to humans.

B-15 also is known as pangamic acid, a name originated by Ernest Krebs, Sr. and Jr., in 1949 for a substance or mixture obtained from rice, barley, or other plants. No one is sure of the exact nature of pangamic acid, probably because it is not a single chemical substance capable of being purified and analyzed. One source describes it as dimethylglycine, another as an ester of gluconic acid and dimethylglycine, yet another as a mixture of diisopropylammonium dichloroacetate, sodium gluconate, and glycine. It is apparent that there is no official standard of identity for this product.

The FDA has seized "vitamin B-15" products, claiming that the claims for it are false and misleading, that it is neither a vitamin nor a provitamin, and that there is no accepted evidence that it has any medical, nutritional or anticancer properties. Both the FDA and the Canadian Food and Drug Directorate have banned the distribution of pangamic acid as a food supplement.

Despite the lack of any published scientific data to validate the clinical use of pangamic acid, a variety of B-15 products remain on the market. The FDA believes these to be potentially dangerous to humans because they contain chemicals that have been shown to lower blood pressure, decrease body temperature, or cause hind-limb paralysis in laboratory test animals. Recently, investigators have reported that when the dimethylglycine ingredient in many "vitamin B-15" products is incubated with sodium nitrate and a substance similar to saliva, the resulting product shows evidence of being cancer-causing.

See also QUACKERY

Vitamin C

Other name: ascorbic acid

Source: citrus fruits; also made synthetically

Pharmacology: prevents clinical signs of scurvy (bleeding gums, loose teeth, muscle weakness, loss of appetite, little hemorrhages in the skin or nose, delayed healing of wounds)

Dose: 60 mg a day is recommended dietary allowance, Food and Nutrition Board, National Academy of Sciences

Well known by its other name, ascorbic acid, vitamin C has been the center of a controversy since famed Nobel laureate Linus Pauling suggested that humans require many thousands of milligrams of it each day to stay healthy, avoid cancer, and live 25 years longer, on the average—this in spite of the medical establishment's recommended dietary allowance of 60 mg a day, an amount clearly sufficient to prevent any clinical sign of scurvy.

Pauling, a world-renowned chemist, now personally ingests 16–18 g of vitamin C daily for "optimum health." His claims that megavitamin C will reduce the number of colds people get, or reduce the severity of symptoms during a cold, have not been substantiated by research tests. Pauling says that the tests were poorly designed. His claim that megavitamin C can improve survival rates in certain cancer patients has not been substantiated by research trials at the Mayo Clinic. Pauling's assertion that high doses of vitamin C will increase life expectancy up to 35 years remains unsubstantiated (Pauling himself is living to a very ripe old age).

Can very large doses of vitamin C be harmful? In most people, probably not. A few high-dosers may experience diarrhea, but usually this is not a major problem. In a few others there may be an increased risk of kidney stone formation; if you have a history of renal calculi, consult your physician before megadosing on vitamin C.

Misuse potential: low

Adverse effects: Doses of vitamin C in the range of 5–10 g a day can cause diarrhea in some people. There is some evidence that kidney stones are more likely to form if you are taking very high doses of vitamin C.

Drug interactions: High blood levels of ascorbic acid are

known to interfere with clinical tests for sugar and steroids in the urine, for cholesterol in the blood, and for blood in the stool. When you plan to have laboratory tests, let your doctor know if you are taking large doses of vitamin C.

Vitamin D

Other names: antirachitic factor, calciferol, irradiated ergosterol, activated ergosterol, ergocalciferol

Sources: fish liver oils, vitamin-fortified milk, synthesized in skin with UV light from food precursors

Pharmacology: prevents rickets; promotes calcium uptake in bone

Dose: Recommended dietary allowance is 400 I.U. for all ages and both sexes.

Hypervitaminosis is a condition of illness due to overdosing on a vitamin. Cases of hypervitaminosis D have been seen in recent years as some people overdo a good thing, prompted especially by advertising aimed at making money rather than curing real deficiencies.

Too much vitamin D can result in calcification (calcium depositing in tissues where we don't want it), kidney stones and kidney damage, retarded physical and mental growth in children, constipation, weakness, stiffness, and high blood pressure. Vitamin D is now considered to be a potent steroidal hormone that clearly can be toxic in high doses. It is easy to overdose on vitamin D because some products are being sold that contain 1000 I.U. per dose.

Vitamin D has been used inappropriately in doses of up to 100,000 I.U. a day for cold hands and feet after thyroidectomy, for arthritis, and for psoriasis.

Beware of urgings of dealers and advertisers to purchase expensive, high-strength vitamin preparations that will automatically make you feel better and more full of energy. You probably will never have to take any vitamin preparation if you consume a balanced diet consisting of the 4 essential food groups: grains, dairy products, vegetables, and meats.

Vitamin E

Other name: tocopherols

Source: widely prevalent in our foods, especially in vegetable oils, fresh greens, and vegetables

Pharmacology: apparently functions as an antoxidant in the body

Dose: not clearly established; probably 10–15 mg per day for adults. NOTE: One milligram of alpha-tocopherol equals 1 I.U.

The role of vitamin E in the human body and our daily requirement for it are not clearly established. In the rat, a deficiency of vitamin E leads to sterility or to testicular degeneration, but no similar findings have been reported in humans.

There is a common belief among the laity that vitamin E is the "sex vitamin" that will increase potency and decrease sterility. Others believe that vitamin E is useful for preventing or treating heart disease. Food quacks and charlatans have promoted these erroneous beliefs and have made a great deal of money from them. The truth is that while we probably need 10–15 mg of vitamin E a day (which we easily get from a varied diet), the 100–1000 mg a day that the food charlatans promote will not prevent or cure any kind of heart disease, sexual impotence, muscle cramp, or other inadequacy.

Misuse potential: medium. Health food stores advertise vitamin E as a nutritional supplement needed in doses of 1000 I.U. or more each day. There is no scientific evidence for such a claim.

Adverse effects: Too much vitamin E is bad for you. At doses of 600 I.U. a day for 8 weeks, it can increase the level of cholesterol in the blood. Some researchers believe that vitamin E is an active drug, not a benign vitamin.

Vivarin

Other name of active ingredient: caffeine

Source: compounding

Pharmacology: Caffeine is a brain and spinal cord stimulant, heart muscle stimulant, cerebral vasoconstrictor, diuretic, and treatment for migraine.

Dose: as a mental stimulant, 1 tablet (200 mg) every 3–4 hours

Knowing that caffeine is a fairly powerful CNS stimulant and that Americans like to experience its effects, pill manufacturers have included caffeine in many OTC products. Each Vivarin tablet contains 200 mg of caffeine; that is considered a heavy dose, and is roughly equivalent to 2 cups of freshly brewed coffee. Caffeine also is found in tea, cola beverages, and chocolate. (See the section on caffeine for amounts contained in these sources.)

In some people caffeine does not seem to have much of an effect. In others it is a potent drug, acting to stimulate the brain and spinal cord, heart, vascular system, and kidneys. Because Vivarin tablets contain the large 200-mg dose and because they are so readily available over-the-counter, it is easy to overdose on this drug. In fact, the manufacturer's recommended dose of 1 tablet every 3–4 hours could mean as much as a gram of caffeine in a day. In sensitive people that will cause insomnia, irregular heartbeat, and fine tremors of the hands, not to mention irritability and headache.

Misuse potential: medium

Adverse effects: Several consumer groups believe that caffeine can cause birth defects; the FDA has not accepted this view. Just the same, you would be wise to restrict your caffeine intake while pregnant. If you exceed the recommended dosage (and sometimes even if you don't), you may experience anxiety, nervousness, wakefulness, and heart palpitations. A dose of 10 g or more of caffeine can cause convulsions. Get medical help immediately if overdosage has occurred.

Drug interactions: Caffeine may raise blood sugar levels, interfering with a diabetic's regular dose of insulin. If you are taking any drug for a heart or kidney condition, see your doctor before taking this product.

See also CAFFEINE

W

WD-40

Other name of main ingredient: petroleum distillates
Source: crude oil
Purported pharmacology: arthritis cure
Dose: applied externally
WD-40 is a maintenance product designed to loosen rusty bolts or stop squeaks; it contains hydrocarbon lubricants made from crude oil. Somehow, WD-40 has gotten the reputation of being an arthritis treatment, but this is utterly ridiculous. The San Diego company that makes WD-40 cautions that it should not be used for any medicinal purpose and should not be applied to the skin. The Arthritis Foundation states that WD-40 has no therapeutic value and that postponing the use of conventional medical treatment could permit the disease to proceed to the crippling stage.
Misuse potential: great
Adverse effects: Applied to the skin, WD-40 can cause dryness and irritation. Swallowing the product can cause nausea, vomiting, and diarrhea; inhaling it can cause a form of pneumonia.
See also QUACKERY

Withdrawal

Other names: withdrawal syndrome, abstinence syndrome, physical withdrawal
When an addict who is physically dependent on a drug is abruptly deprived of any amount of it, he or she will enter a period of physical and mental agitation known as a withdrawal

syndrome. The withdrawal episode can be mild, with only nervousness, slight tremor, or a runny nose. Or it can be very traumatic: nausea, vomiting, tremors, hallucinations, intestinal spasm, back pain, diarrhea, uncontrollable orgasm, or life-threatening convulsions.

Abrupt withdrawal from alcohol, barbiturates, opiates, or Valium can be very serious, even life-threatening; withdrawal from nicotine or caffeine, much less so. NOTE: To experience physical withdrawal one has to be addicted physically, not just psychologically dependent. In true physical dependency, changes occur in the body so that the person needs the drug as a "normal" part of life. In withdrawal, this "normalcy" is being challenged and the body is being reset to function without the drug once again.

The problem is that most heavy drug users do not realize they are becoming physically addicted or dependent. The user of alcohol or Valium, Demerol, barbiturates, or other prescription sleeping pills may gradually build up the dose over many months or years. Insidiously, frequent use leads to habituation; habituation becomes preoccupation; preoccupation becomes compulsive use and finally physical addiction or psychological dependence. The greater risk factors are the type of drug and the size and frequency of dose. Sleeping pills, tranquilizers, and painkillers have high abuse potential, and the more drug you take and the more often you take it, the more likely you are to develop a dependence on it, especially if you have a history of drug misuse (such as increasing doses on your own initiative). If you understand this, you will understand the advice about taking the smallest dose of the drug that will accomplish the desired effect, and for the briefest period. Certainly, a sleeping pill should not be used more than 1 or 2 nights—never for a week or longer. The best advice is not to take the drug in the first place!

Drugs such as cocaine or marijuana do not lead to physical dependence in the doses typically used. However, it is now generally accepted that very heavy use (large daily doses) of either cocaine or marijuana can lead to a physical addiction with a withdrawal syndrome. Very high plasma levels of these drugs are required before this can happen.

The acute, physical phase of withdrawal can last as long as 5 days. Since the agony can be ended at any time by readministering the drug, there is a great temptation for the addict to take another dose. Secondary withdrawals are known. Valium addicts, for example, can experience withdrawal symptoms for up to 2 years after the last dose (see the section on Valium).

Withdrawal can be accomplished "cold turkey" in a hotel room, in jail, or in a hospital with medical assistance. Withdrawal from a full-fledged addiction to Valium, other benzodiazepine tranquilizers, Valmid, barbiturates, or other sleeping pills can involve life-threatening convulsions. Do not attempt such a withdrawal on your own; seek medical assistance. Sometimes other drugs are prescribed to ease the physical and mental anguish of withdrawal. However, great care must be taken to avoid the development of a secondary dependence, as has happened when the minor tranquilizer Serax was used in alcohol detoxifications.

NOTE: Not all heroin abusers experience serious withdrawal syndromes when they stop taking their drug. Some heroin users are of the weekend variety; they are called "chippers." Their main symptoms when they detoxify are a runny nose and maybe some flulike symptoms.

See also ADDICTION, NARCOTIC ANALGESICS

Wyanoids Suppositories

Other names for main ingredients: belladonna extract, ephedrine
Source: compounding
Pharmacology: hemorrhoid treatment
Dose: 1 suppository twice daily for 6 days

This product, sold as a treatment for hemorrhoids, contains belladonna extract, ephedrine, zinc oxide, boric acid, bismuth oxyiodide, bismuth subcarbonate, Peruvian balsam, and cocoa butter. There is also an ointment form that contains benzocaine (local anesthetic), boric acid, zinc oxide (protectant), Peruvian balsam, castor oil, petrolatum, and ephedrine.

These are the worst examples of "shotgun" formulations; they contain a great many ingredients in the hope that something will do some good. The FDA has concluded that this product lacks evidence of safety and effectiveness in at least 1 ingredient, the combination of ingredients, or the dosage form.

Misuse potential: high. Suppositories, though widely advertised, have proven to be of little value for relieving the pain of hemorrhoids. When inserted, the suppository usually passes by the painful area and melts farther into the rectum. If there is bleeding from a varicose vein, the suppository cannot be relied upon to stop it. Any rectal bleeding should be treated by a physician, not with a suppository. You may be able to get more pain relief by sitting in a warm bath or lying down. After a bowel movement, gentle cleansing of the anal area with lukewarm water can be helpful.

Adverse effects: Wyanoids suppositories contain belladonna alkaloids; these are potent drugs that can affect the heart and other organs. Use of this product can worsen glaucoma (a too-high pressure in the eyeballs, often seen in the elderly). If you experience rapid heartbeat, dizziness, blurred vision, or dryness of the mouth, discontinue use of this product. If you use this product and feel pain in your eye, discontinue use and see a doctor immediately, as you may have undiagnosed glaucoma.

Drug interactions: Antipsychotic drugs such as Mellaril, Thorazine, and Trilafon and the antihistamine Benadryl have actions similar to those of the belladonna alkaloids; these drugs can add to the anticholinergic action of the belladonna alkaloids contained in these suppositories. Monoamine oxidase inhibitors such as Parnate and Nardil can increase the actions of ephedrine in the body.

See also HEMORRHOIDAL PRODUCTS

X

XTC (Ecstasy). *See* HALLUCINOGENIC AMPHETAMINE DERIVATIVES

Y

Yohimbine

Other names: Yocon, Yohimex, yohimbine alkaloid
Source: plant
Pharmacology: alpha-2 adrenergic blocker; hallucinogen; purported aphrodisiac
Dose: variable

The main source of yohimbine is the yohimbehe bark from a tree that is native to Africa. The substance has been sold illegally as an aphrodisiac ("passion pill"). Promoters cite a single Canadian hospital study in which 23 sexually unresponsive people were given yohimbine for 10 weeks. Six of the 23 responded with arousal. Yohimbine is now available in the United States as the prescription drugs Yocon and Yohimex. Medical researchers have identified yohimbine as an alpha-2 adrenergic blocking agent useful in the treatment and diagnostic classification of some types of male erectile impotence. It can also be used as a mydriatic (agent that dilates the pupil of the eye).

Abuse potential: high

Adverse effects: Yohimbine was identified 25 years ago as a hallucinogen of the indolethylamine type (a category that also includes LSD and psylocin). It was found to raise heart rate and blood pressure, and to be a powerful stimulant to anxiety, as well as an activator of schizophrenic psychosis. Subjects who took it became tense, irritable, restless, and anxious. Yohimbine does not appear to be a safe substance for casual use; in doses of 30–40 mg it appears capable of causing undesirable psychological effects. (The dose of yohimbine in Yocon and Yohimex tablets is 5.4 and 5.0 mg, respectively.) CAUTION: Do not use yohimbine-containing drugs during pregnancy or if you suffer from kidney disease.

Drug interactions: Simultaneous use of other brain stimulants such as epinephrine will add to the effects of yohimbine.

Yucca

Other name: none

Source: plant

Pharmacology: purported arthritis treatment

Yucca is a herbal extract from a cactus plant; it has been used by Indians of the Southwest for many years to treat sore joints. Recently a clinic in Southern California has promoted yucca as a treatment for arthritis, claiming that the substance is a hormone that passes through the digestive tract unabsorbed, improving digestion and eliminating wastes and toxins.

There is no scientific evidence to support the claim that yucca has any effect on the underlying causes of arthritis.

Misuse potential: high

Adverse effects: The major problem with the use of unproven concoctions such as yucca is the uncertainty of what you are ingesting. Are there any harmful ingredients in the extract? Has the bacterial content been checked? Is it safe to take the product repeatedly over a period of days or weeks? If there are adverse effects to a substance such as yucca, you might be the "guinea pig" who would discover them.

Glossary

active ingredient The specific chemical in a drug or plant that is responsible for the drug action ascribed to the entire preparation.

agonist A drug that stimulates a receptor to produce a pharmacological effect. Contrast with antagonist.

analgesic Relieving pain.

ANS Autonomic nervous system. Nerves in the body that control involuntary or independent functions.

antagonist A drug that binds to a receptor, producing no action of its own, thereby blocking the action of an agonist.

anticholinergic A drug that blocks nerve conduction through parasympathetic nerves or inhibits the actions of acetylcholine. Atropine is the quintessential anticholinergic drug.

antihypertensive Reducing a too-high blood pressure.

antipsychotic A drug for the treatment of psychotic states, including schizophrenia.

antipyretic A drug that lowers an elevated body temperature; an antifever drug.

antitussive A cough suppressant.

benzodiazepine A chemical category to which many of the minor tranquilizers belong.

beta-blocker A drug that inhibits or blocks the actions of drugs on beta-adrenergic receptors—for example, in the heart.

blood-brain barrier The fatlike barrier separating the blood from the cerebrospinal fluid.

blood sugar Glucose, the sugar normally found in the blood. Also known as dextrose.

catecholamines Neurotransmitters in the body having the dihydroxy-phenethylamine chemical structure. Examples are epinephrine and norepinephrine.

cholinergic Nerves that use acetylcholine as their synaptic transmitter.

CNS   Central nervous system, consisting of the brain and spinal column.

controlled substance   A drug or chemical regulated under the federal Controlled Substances Act of 1970. Its manufacture, distribution, and sale are subject to federal control or punishment. The key criterion for controlling a substance is its potential for abuse and dependence.

DAWN   Drug Abuse Warning Network, operated by the federal government.

DEA   Drug Enforcement Administration

diuretic   An agent that increases the flow of urine.

drug fever   Fever induced by a drug, often as part of an allergic response to the drug.

electrolytes   Minerals in the blood or elsewhere that are ionized (carry an electrical charge). They contribute to osmotic effects. In the laboratory they cause the solution to carry an electrical charge.

endocrine system   All the glands that secrete hormones.

enteric-coated   Covered or coated with a special substance that prevents dissolving until the intestine is reached. Used for drugs that would irritate the stomach.

enzyme   A biological chemical, protein in nature, produced by living cells, and that can influence the rate of body processes. Enzymes can act independently of the cells that produce them.

estrogen   A female sex hormone; responsible for secondary sex characteristics.

FDA   The U.S. Food and Drug Administration, a branch of the U.S. Department of Health and Human Services.

FSH   Follicle-stimulating hormone.

g   The gram. A unit of mass in the metric system. One pound is 454 g.

GI   Gastrointestinal—that is, referring to the stomach and the intestines.

gonadotropin   A hormone secreted by the pituitary gland that stimulates the gonads (ovaries and testes).

half-life   The time (usually expressed in hours) required for half the dose of a drug to be excreted from the body.

hypnotic   A drug or substance that induces sleep.

IM   Intramuscularly. A drug can be injected IM.

inflammation   A defense body process characterized by redness, heat, pain, and swelling, and caused by injury to tissue.

IU   International Unit. Used to measure doses of drugs or biologicals.

IV   Intravenous. A drug can be injected IV. On the street such a route is termed mainlining.

kg Kilogram. A unit of mass in the metric system. One kg equals 1000 g, or 2.2 pounds.

libido Sex drive.

lipid A fat or fatlike substance.

mainline (a drug) Inject intravenously.

metabolism (of drugs) All the chemical and physical reactions the body carries out to transform a drug or prepare it for excretion.

metabolite In the broad sense, any substance produced by the body as a result of normal functioning. Specifically, a breakdown product of a drug that may or may not have activity itself.

mg Milligram. One one-thousandth of a gram.

mg/kg Dosage. A method of calculating the size of a dose based on the mass of the patient, not age. If the drug company determines the dose to 1 mg/kg and the patient weighs 70 kg (154 pounds), the dose would be 70 mg.

ml Milliliter. One one-thousandth of a liter. Also written mL. Approximately 30 ml equal 1 fluid ounce.

narcotic A drug that relieves pain and simultaneously depresses the CNS; in large enough doses it produces stupor. Narcotic analgesic usually is inferred.

neuroleptic A major tranquilizing drug used to treat psychotic episodes.

neurotransmitter A chemical released from the end of one nerve to carry the nerve impulse across the synapse to the next nerve.

ng Nanogram. One-billionth of a gram.

orthostatic hypotension Dizziness or fainting upon abrupt standing, owing to fall in blood pressure as blood drains away from the head.

OTC Over-the-counter. Legally purchasable without a prescription.

parasympathetic The division of the autonomic nervous system that deals with activities that conserve and restore body energy and eliminate body waste.

parenteral Giving a drug by any route of injection.

P.D.R. *Physicians' Desk Reference.* A well-known book in which drug companies list their products along with descriptions, actions, warnings, drug interactions, adverse effects, dosage, and so forth. One edition covers prescription-only drugs; the other, non-prescription drugs.

peristalsis The wavelike contractions of the GI tract by which the contents are propelled along.

pharmacology The science that deals with the sources, actions, side effects, adverse effects, distribution, and fate of drugs in animal organisms.

platelets Normal constituents of the blood, smaller than red cells, and essential to the process of blood clotting.

pressor drug One that will raise blood pressure.

prophylactic Warding off disease.

psychoactive Having an effect upon the mind or behavior.

receptor site Specialized cells in a body tissue to which a drug or chemical attaches to exert its pharmacological effect.

REM sleep Rapid-eye-movement sleep, indicating dreaming.

reservoir (drug) Any system, fluid, organ, or part of the body that can bind and hold a drug for an extended period of time, thus delaying its rapid elimination from the body.

SC Subcutaneous. Beneath the skin, as in an injection.

septicemia Blood poisoning. Presence and growth of pathogenic infectious organisms in the blood.

side effect An expected or predictable effect of a drug that accompanies the main, desired effect. Side effects are usually but not always undesirable.

sublingual Under the tongue.

superinfection The development of a secondary infection superimposed upon an initial infection, often due to overgrowth of microorganisms that are normally present. For example, antibiotic therapy may upset the healthy balance of microbes in the intestine or vagina, allowing the nonsusceptible organisms to multiply uncontrolled.

sympathetic A division of the autonomic nervous system that can mobilize the body to handle stressful situations. Tends to discharge as a whole.

synapse The extremely tiny space where one nerve ends and the next begins; site of action of various neurotransmitters.

syndrome All the signs and symptoms associated with a disease.

teratogen A drug or agent capable of causing birth defects by its action upon the embryo or fetus.

tolerance Resistance to a drug acquired after prolonged use; necessitates taking an ever larger dose to obtain the same effect.

toxicity The poisonous character of a substance. Acute and chronic aspects are recognized.

U.S.P. *United States Pharmacopoeia.* An official compendium and reference book for drugs used in the United States.

withdrawal syndrome A crisis, with varying degrees of physical and emotional severity, that can accompany the abrupt removal of a drug on which the person has become dependent.